Ready or Not?

Ready or Not?

A Girl's Guide to Making
Her Own Decisions About Dating,
Love, and Sex

Tina Radziszewicz

Illustrated by Kathryn Lamb

Walker & Company · New York

Published in the United States of America in 2006 by
Walker Publishing Company, Inc.
Distributed to the trade by Holtzbrinck Publishers

First published in Great Britain in 2005 by Piccadilly Press Ltd.

For information about permission to reproduce selections from
this book, write to Permissions, Walker & Company,
104 Fifth Avenue, New York, New York 10011

Library of Congress Cataloging-in-Publication Data
Radziszewicz, Tina.
Ready or not? : A girl's guide to making her own decisions about dating,
love, and sex / Tina Radziszewicz ; illustrations by Kathryn Lamb.
        p.   cm.
Includes index.
ISBN-10: 0-8027-9613-3 • ISBN-13: 978-0-8027-9613-4 (hardcover)
ISBN-10: 0-8027-9612-5 • ISBN-13: 978-0-8027-9612-7 (paperback)
1. Sex instruction for girls. 2. Dating (Social customs). 3. Teenage pregnancy—
Prevention. 4. Sexually transmitted diseases—Prevention. I. Title.
HQ51.R35 2006   613.9071′2—dc22   2006016891

Visit Walker & Company's Web site at www.walkeryoungreaders.com

Printed in the U.S.A. by Quebecor World Fairfield
2 4 6 8 10 9 7 5 3 1

This book is dedicated to my loving and patient family—
Mark (especially!), Daniel and Dorothy, Alex, Oscar and Fatty—
and those in the next room—Chris, Waclaw and Irene.
Thanks also to the readers of bliss *magazine, past and present,*
without whose insights this book would never have been written.

CONTENTS

Hello and Welcome to Your Book!   x

Using This Book   xi

PART ONE: YOUR BODY AND YOU

Chapter One: Puberty   3

Growing Up   3

Your Body   5

His Body   15

Chapter Two: Periods   21

Your Internal Reproductive System   21

Your Period   24

Chapter Three: Here's Looking at You   36

Body Image   36

Eating Disorders   41

Boobs   44

Quiz: Body Language   50

Body Positive   53

Chapter Four: Body Q & A   57

PART TWO: EMOTIONS AND YOU

Chapter Five: The Dating Game   67

Attraction   68

Quiz: Boy Gauge—What's He After?   73

Dating   75

Having a Boyfriend   77

Chapter Six: Sexuality   84

Common Questions About Sexuality   85

Masturbation   89
Gay or Straight?   92

Chapter Seven: Attitudes Toward Sex   95
Parents   96
Religion and Culture   98
The Media   99
Friends   100
School   100
Sex and the Law   101
Your Values   104

Chapter Eight: Emotions Q & A   105

PART THREE: SEX AND YOU

Chapter Nine: Are You Ready for Sex?   115
Virginity   116
Waiting to Have Sex   117
Right Time, Right Person   118
Questions to Ask Yourself   119
Bad Reasons for Having Sex   122
Regrets   123

Chapter Ten: Contraception   125
Contraception: What's It All About?   125
Methods of Contraception   129
Emergency Contraception   151

Chapter Eleven: Sexually Transmitted Diseases and
      Women's Health   156
STDs: What's What   160
Women's Health   174

Chapter Twelve: Boys and Sex   180
The Differences Between Boys and Girls   180

Name-Calling   185
Boys' Top Ten Tales to Get You into Bed   187
Boys and Girls on Dates   192

Chapter Thirteen: Let's Talk About Sex   193
Parents   193
Friends   197
Boyfriends   199
Doctors and Other Health Professionals   206

Chapter Fourteen: Test Your Sexpertise   211
Quiz: Are You a Sexpert?   211

Chapter Fifteen: Having Sex   214
Before Sexual Intercourse   214
Having Sexual Intercourse   217
Sex Myths Exposed   222

Chapter Sixteen: Sex—When You Don't Want It   224
Sexual Harassment   225
Sexual Abuse   226
Sexual Assault   230
Rape   230
Sexual Assault and Alcohol   234
What to Do if You've Been Sexually Assaulted or Raped   234
Feelings After a Sexual Attack   236
Helping a Friend Who's Been Attacked   237
Staying Safe   238

Chapter Seventeen: Getting Pregnant   242
Are You Pregnant?   243
Your Options   247

Chapter Eighteen: Your Most Embarrassing Sex
                    Questions Answered   252

Resources and Contacts   259
Acknowledgments   268
Index   269

HELLO AND WELCOME
TO YOUR BOOK!

Having read thousands of your letters during my years as an advice columnist, I know how hard finding out information on sex and relationships can be for teenagers. So I was really pleased to be asked to write this book. At last I can give you the answers to your questions on boys, bodies, relationships, and sex—all in one place.

There are tons of myths and rumors about sex, ranging from the plain silly to the downright harmful, and this book is intended to give you the facts.

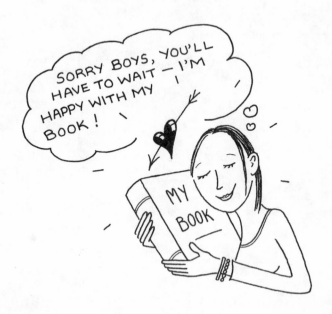

USING THIS BOOK

Of course, you can flip through and check out the stuff that's caught your eye, but I've arranged the book so that each chapter covers what you need to know in roughly the order each issue will crop up if you're starting to think about sexual relationships. You'll find plenty of advice and reassurance, plus contact details for further help, throughout the pages, as well as a comprehensive "Resources and Contacts" section at the end.

Whatever stage you're at, in order to stay safe from pregnancy, sexually transmitted diseases, and some of the emotional difficulties of sex (such as feeling under pressure to do stuff you're not ready for), you can never know too much. So if you want to be educated and sensible about sex, this is the book for you.

Tina Radziszewicz

PART ONE

Your Body and You

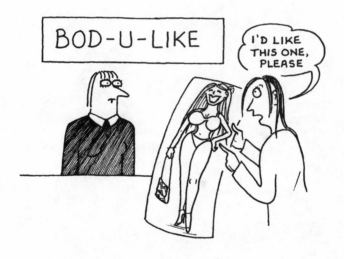

CHAPTER ONE
Puberty

Welcome to the first chapter. Even if you're over puberty, read on, anyway. Going over the basics of your bod and his will put the rest of the book in context, and you never know—you might learn something!

Chapter 1 covers:

- Growing Up
- Your Body: Shape, Height, and Appearance; Boobs; Body Hair; Skin and Hair; Sweat; Your Genitals; Your Orgasm
- His Body: Shape, Height, and Appearance; Skin and Hair; Sweat; Voice; His Genitals; His Orgasm

GROWING UP

Just before I started writing this book, I got the following letter:

I'm fifteen, and I'm the only girl in my class with a flat chest. I've liked this cute boy for two years and gotten up the courage to text him, but he never replied. My friends say the fact that I'm pimply and taller than most of the boys probably put him off. I've never even kissed anyone and I'm terrified I'll never get a boyfriend. I'm so depressed. Please help!

Becky, 15

Becky's letter made me think back to when I was a teenager. Boob-wise, I had the opposite problem as her, and it was a huge source of worry. My chest swelled to a 34B when I was just eleven. Too young to cope with the unwanted attention and rude comments, I hid in baggy tops for years. And until I was sixteen, I had a complexion that wouldn't have looked out of place on a pizza advertisement. If I'd had straight hair instead of a lopsided Afro, I'd probably have grown chin-length bangs to hide my face.

That's the thing about puberty—everything about you can seem too embarrassing for words. As a kid, your biggest worry is whether you'll get a Mermaid Barbie to add to your collection. Then next thing you know, you're wondering when your period will start and considering removing all the mirrors in your house.

Your mind and body are changing so fast that it can sometimes feel as though everything's wrong. You're too short or too tall, too flat-chested or too busty, and, on top of all that, you've just had a screaming fight with your mom and your crush doesn't know you exist. It seems so unfair when all you want is to be the same as your friends and get noticed by Justin in homeroom.

Puberty and the part that comes after it, adolescence, is the period when you change from a child into an adult. For girls, Mother Nature's grand plan is to equip their bodies to produce babies. Similarly for boys, the main goal is to make them capable of becoming fathers. How ironic that so many of us spend most of our lives trying to avoid pregnancy!

Puberty starts at around ten or eleven in girls, and by seventeen or so, you'll have reached your adult height and shape. For some, puberty and being a teenager feels like a nonstop roller coaster of ever-changing emotions, new sexual feelings, and physical changes, but others aren't necessarily stomping off in a bad mood every two minutes, and some actually find their teen years to be one of the most enjoyable periods of their lives. After all, there's a lot of new, exciting stuff going on—first date, first kiss, first sexual experiences. You're learning to be independent of your parents, changing schools, making more friends, and thinking about your future.

But whether you're ticked off with life like Becky, more chilled than a penguin's butt, or somewhere in between, you're bound to have questions. Knowledge, as they say, is power, so if you understand what's going on with your body, you'll find it a bit easier to take a step back and be patient with yourself.

YOUR BODY

Puberty is controlled by an increase in chemicals called hormones, and these affect your mind as well as your body. For girls, it's the female sex hormones estrogen and progesterone that kick in at ten or eleven, or it could be a year or so later or earlier than this. A bit of pubic hair or your boobs beginning to swell are usually the first signs that puberty has started. Periods tend to come later on, at around eleven to fourteen, after your internal sexual organs have matured. Your voice will also get a bit deeper as your voice box grows, but this is so gradual that you may not notice.

Not everyone experiences these changes at the same time, so try not to panic if you're developing more quickly or slowly than your friends. Everyone's body has its own timetable.

Shape, Height, and Appearance

You'll shoot up in height and might even tower over the boys in your grade for a while. Girls start developing a couple of years earlier than boys, although the boys gradually catch up and, you won't be surprised to hear, generally end up taller than girls. Your face shape will change too, with your jaw and nose becoming more defined and the space between your eyes and hairline increasing. Your weight will almost double over the seven or so years it takes to develop your adult shape, but it's worth it because you get boobs and a waist that's narrower in relation to your curvy hips.

Lots of girls feel alarmed by their new, more rounded shape in a culture that seems to value thinness. Worries about body image and how you look are important areas that we'll tackle in more detail in chapter 3.

Boobs

When your boobs first start developing, your nipples will stick out while the rest of your breasts stay flat. You might find that your nipples tingle a little from time to time, which is due to the growth process. Boobs are made up of fatty tissue containing tiny glands that produce milk if you have a baby. We all have the same number of milk-producing glands, but some girls have more fat up top than others, which is why their breasts are bigger. It's also common for one boob to end up larger than the other. For more on breasts, see chapter 3.

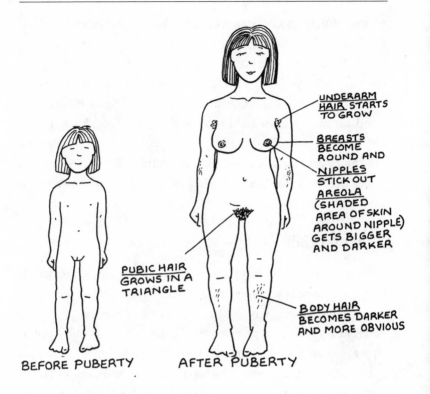

UNDERARM HAIR STARTS TO GROW

BREASTS BECOME ROUND AND

NIPPLES STICK OUT

AREOLA (SHADED AREA OF SKIN AROUND NIPPLE) GETS BIGGER AND DARKER

PUBIC HAIR GROWS IN A TRIANGLE

BODY HAIR BECOMES DARKER AND MORE OBVIOUS

BEFORE PUBERTY   AFTER PUBERTY

Body Hair

You'll get hair under your arms and on your pubic area, and possibly one or two strands around your nipples. Plus the hair on your arms and legs will become thicker, particularly on your legs. Many girls like to shave their legs or get them waxed, especially in summer. In general, shaving your armpits is easier than waxing. Some people believe that removing hair makes it grow back faster, but it's not true.

Some girls end up with a small amount of pale pubic hair, while others get darker, coarser hair that can spread to the top

7

of their thighs and even creep up toward their stomach. Hair that's visible at the edges of your panty legs is known as your bikini line, and some girls like to remove this. It's not a good idea to shave your bikini line, particularly if you have coarse, curly hair, as you may have a problem with ingrown hairs and wind up with red, itchy bumps as the hair grows back. If you can't afford a professional waxing, you can buy wax at the pharmacy and do it yourself. Although this can be tricky, it gets easier the more you do it. Waxing or hair-removing creams are best for the bikini line and last longer.

Skin and Hair

During puberty in boys *and* girls, it's the male hormone testosterone that's responsible for the increase in sebum (a fancy name for oil), which can lead to greasy skin and pimples. Nearly everyone gets pimples from time to time. It's best not to squeeze them, as you can end up with scars, but if your skin gets really bad, ask your doctor if one of the many effective prescription drugs is right for you. Over-the-counter preparations containing benzoyl peroxide can help mild acne, although some people find it dries out their skin. It's important to include five portions of fruit and veggies in your daily diet for your general health, although what we eat (including chocolate!) has little effect on acne because the main culprit is the male sex hormone.

Your hair will probably get greasier too. Don't brush or comb it too much because this will stimulate your glands to produce more oil. Wash it daily with a small amount of mild shampoo, and beware conditioner—best leave it alone if your hair's very greasy or you'll end up looking like you've slept on an oil slick.

Sweat

As the sweat glands in your armpits start to work, you'll need to use something to control perspiration. Sweat is how the body cools itself down as the water on your skin evaporates. Fresh sweat doesn't smell, but after a while, bacteria get to work and *then*, well, you know about it! It's best to bathe or shower daily. Deodorants are made to disguise the smell of sweat, while antiperspirants reduce the amount you sweat. Hair traps sweat and makes you more likely to smell in the hairier parts of your body. But it's up to you whether you remove the hair under your arms or not.

The sweat glands in your genital area also become active. Just like your underarms, some people sweat more than others down below. If it bothers you, don't go for the powders and sprays on the market for your "intimate" area, as the chemicals can cause irritation. A good swish around once a day (maybe more in summer) with unperfumed soap is all you need—with, of course, a daily change of underwear.

Your Genitals

Although some people refer to the whole area between a girl's legs as her vagina, the correct name for this area is the vulva. (We'll come to the vagina later.)

Plenty is changing here too. If you've never had a look at your genital region before, now might be a good time to grab yourself a mirror. Some girls think it's weird or yucky to look at themselves, but it's your body and it's a good idea to get to know it. And it makes tampon insertion a whole lot easier if you know what you're aiming for.

Here's a diagram to help you, but don't expect your vulva to look exactly like this. Genital appearance varies hugely, just as faces do.

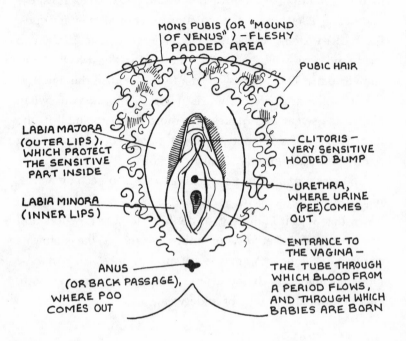

MONS PUBIS (OR "MOUND OF VENUS") – FLESHY PADDED AREA

PUBIC HAIR

LABIA MAJORA (OUTER LIPS), WHICH PROTECT THE SENSITIVE PART INSIDE

CLITORIS – VERY SENSITIVE HOODED BUMP

LABIA MINORA (INNER LIPS)

URETHRA, WHERE URINE (PEE) COMES OUT

ANUS (OR BACK PASSAGE), WHERE POO COMES OUT

ENTRANCE TO THE VAGINA – THE TUBE THROUGH WHICH BLOOD FROM A PERIOD FLOWS, AND THROUGH WHICH BABIES ARE BORN

Mons Pubis

Also known as the Mound of Venus (which is pretty nice, Venus being the goddess of love and all that), the mons pubis is the cushiony area where your legs meet that's covered in hair by the time puberty is complete. It protects the place where your pubic bones join and, when you become sexually active, acts as a bumper during sexual intercourse when your partner is on top.

Labia Majora

This means large lips, and they're the fleshy outer ones you come to first. They protect the inner areas and keep moisture in. During puberty, they get thicker and darker and also become covered in hair.

Labia Minora

It won't surprise you to hear that these are the small lips, and they're visible when you part the labia majora. In some girls, they're hidden by the outer lips, while in others, they hang down between them. Or you might have one longer than the other—it's all normal. These inner lips are moist and hairless and, the darker your skin, the darker in color they are, so they can range from pale pink to dark brown. They join at the top to form the hood of the clitoris.

Clitoris

People used to think the vagina was the main source of sexual stimulation for women, but we now know that most women find it's the clitoris that's crucial to their orgasm (the peak of sexual pleasure). Just peeping out from its hood, the clitoris is made of the same tissue as the penis. It has loads of nerve endings and is therefore very sensitive, as you'll discover if you touch it. Like the penis, it fills with blood and lots of girls find it becomes firm when they're sexually aroused, although, being a lot smaller than a penis, it's not as noticeable.

Urethra

Below your clitoris is your urethra, the tiny opening that you pee from, which leads to your bladder through a short tube. It's completely separate from your vagina, as you saw in the diagram, and is far too small for the penis to fit into, which some girls worry about needlessly.

Vagina

The vagina isn't a hole. It's a hollow, muscular tube with flexible walls that can stretch to accommodate a penis or tampon and, when and if you get around to it, a baby. It's normally wet with a whitish fluid that contains lots of friendly bacteria and keeps the vagina clean. Before puberty, the vagina is shorter and its walls are thinner, which is why it can cause damage if a girl has sex before her body has developed.

Normally the walls touch each other like a collapsed balloon. When you're sexually excited, more blood flows into the area and your vagina lengthens at the top end to accommodate a penis. Fluid filters in from the walls, lubricating the vagina so that it's easier for a penis to slide in.

Rather than going straight back, your vagina angles upward. At the top of it is the neck of your womb (the cervix), which feels like the tip of your nose with a dimple in the center. This dimple is a small hole (the os), the entrance to your womb. The os is the diameter of a thin straw—far too small for a penis to enter or a tampon to get lost in. The cervix produces mucus that changes with your menstrual cycle, and becomes thicker if you take birth-control pills.

G-spot

This is named after Dr. Ernst Gräftenberg, the first doctor to describe it. Some sex researchers believe that all women have a G-spot, although gynecologists (specialists who deal with the female reproductive system) haven't been able to locate it. In general, women who say they have one claim they can only feel it when they're sexually aroused. The G-spot is described as a ridged, bean-sized bump in the upper vaginal wall (under the stomach). For some, gentle but firm pressure on this spot produces an orgasm.

Hymen

Most, but not all, girls are born with a thin tissue of skin—the hymen—across the vaginal opening. Hymens vary a great deal. Some cover the vaginal opening completely, but most have holes through which your period can flow. The hymen skin is so thin that it can easily be broken by bike or horseback riding or other vigorous activity, so for the majority of girls, when they first have sex, the hymen is already broken.

If a girl's hymen is intact the first time she has sexual intercourse, she may bleed a little—certainly not enough to need a tampon. Whether your hymen's broken or not, you're a virgin until the first time you have sex.

Your Orgasm

An orgasm is the peak of sexual pleasure, and your body passes through various stages before it happens.

When you start to feel sexually excited, the walls of your vagina secrete droplets of moisture, known as vaginal lubrication. Some girls find they get very wet, while others might not notice anything. As your excitement increases, it's common to feel a tightness or fullness in your genital area. Your nipples may stick out and your breasts swell and become very sensitive. Inside, your womb lifts up and the length of your vagina increases to allow more room for a penis. If your skin's fair, you might notice blotches on your tummy and chest as your blood flow increases. You may start to pant and your legs, arms, stomach, and genitals may feel tense or heavy as your heart begins to thump. This can feel scary if you're not used to it, but in time, you'll learn to relax and go with the feelings.

The next phase is orgasm, but some girls stay at the previous stage, either because they haven't learned to have an orgasm or because they just want to enjoy this feeling of arousal. It can feel uncomfortable and frustrating if you don't have an orgasm. For the majority of girls, orgasm results from stimulation of their clitoris.

The orgasm itself is a series of pleasurable short, rhythmic contractions in the muscles around your vagina, womb, and anus. You may feel warm and tingly all over your body as well. When a boy or girl has had an orgasm, we say they've "come." For boys, coming also means ejaculating (releasing semen from their penis). Most women don't release liquid at orgasm, but some do—and it can be quite a lot. Sex researchers say this liquid comes out of the urethra, but it's definitely not urine. They believe it's made in a gland in front of the bladder. Stimulation of the G-spot is supposed to make this release of liquid, known as female ejaculation, more likely.

After an orgasm, you feel drowsy and relaxed as your body returns to normal. If you were very turned on and didn't come, this process takes longer. For more information on orgasms, see chapters 6 and 15.

HIS BODY

Meanwhile, there's lots going on over in the boy camp at puberty too. For boys, the process starts a little later than for girls—when they're twelve or thirteen, on average, although like girls, it can be earlier or later. The first sign is usually that their testicles (balls) and penis start to grow, and they'll get a few wispy hairs where their penis joins their body and possibly also under their arms.

Shape, Height, and Appearance

The hormone responsible for puberty in boys is the male hormone testosterone (although girls have an increase of testosterone at puberty too). A boy's growth spurt tends to start at twelve or thirteen, but he often won't reach his full adult height and shoulder width until his early twenties. Like girls, boys' weight will also double, although in their case this is mostly muscle. The shape of their face changes too, resulting in a higher forehead and more prominent nose and jaw.

Skin and Hair

Because of their newly oily skin, boys are prone to pimples during puberty too. The hair on boys' legs and arms will get thicker and darker, but much more so than girls'. They may get a hairy belly and chest in their twenties, although some boys remain relatively hairless in those areas. A hairy dad generally means a hairy son. Facial hair appears between thirteen and fifteen on average, and it can be a big source of worry for boys if they're among the last to sprout it.

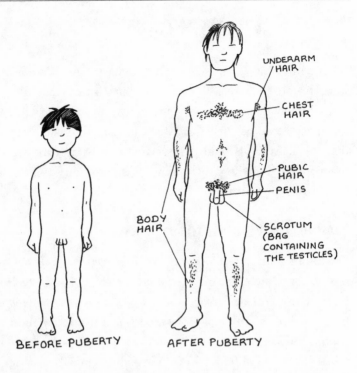

UNDERARM HAIR

CHEST HAIR

PUBIC HAIR

PENIS

BODY HAIR

SCROTUM (BAG CONTAINING THE TESTICLES)

BEFORE PUBERTY   AFTER PUBERTY

Sweat

Like girls, as boys' sweat glands develop, they will need to shower each day and use a deodorant or antiperspirant. Smelly feet tend to be more of a problem for boys, especially if they wear nylon socks and sneakers.

Voice

At about age fourteen, a boy's voice will break. Luckily, nothing actually gets damaged. What happens is that a boy's voice box, or larynx, gets bigger, which is often visible to the outside world as the Adam's apple. The vocal cords inside get thicker and longer, deepening the voice. For some, this happens so slowly that they don't notice their voice changing, while others go through a croaky or squeaky phase and then find they're speaking in huskier tones than before.

His Genitals

Testicles

You might have heard about boys' balls "dropping" as they reach puberty. In fact, the testicles descend gradually from being up inside their body to hanging outside in a loose bag of skin called the scrotum. While their scrotum grows, their penis gets longer and thicker. The skin of the balls and penis darkens, ranging from reddish in fair-skinned boys to shades of brown in those with darker skin. In the same way that girls rarely have equal sized breasts, one testicle usually hangs lower than the other.

Penis

A year or so after the penis has started to lengthen, boys find they can ejaculate (come). This is when a whitish liquid leaks or spurts out during orgasm. Initially, their ejaculations don't contain sperm, but this is only at the beginning stages of puberty.

The penis consists of the head (also called the glans), which, like the girl's clitoris, is very sensitive, and the shaft. The penis is made of spongy tissue that, when a boy is sexually excited, fills with blood, making it harden and stick out from his body (called an erection). Boys ejaculate and pee through a hole in the end of the penis. Tiny muscles at the bladder entrance close it off before ejaculation, making sure they don't release semen and urine at the same time.

The hormones newly coursing around boys' and girls' bodies means that for both of you, sex can be on your mind 24/7. Boys suddenly start getting erections all over the place. These can even happen when an erection is the last thing they want. When hard, penises can point left, straight ahead, or right (sounds like traffic directions, I know), and most have a slight curve.

At some point, nearly all boys worry that their penis is too small. In fact, when erect, most end up measuring between five and seven inches.

Circumcision

Boys are born with a sheath of skin, called the foreskin, covering the head of the penis. In some cultures—for example, Jewish and Muslim—the foreskin is cut away soon after birth, although some Muslim boys get this done later in childhood. A grown man might have his foreskin removed either because he feels it's easier to keep clean that way or because the foreskin is so tight that it can't be pulled back, making sexual intercourse or masturbation very painful. Removal of the foreskin is known as circumcision.

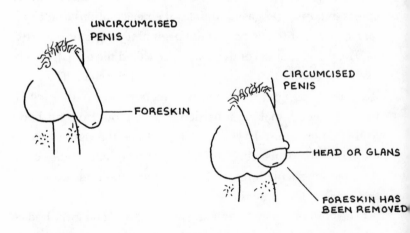

UNCIRCUMCISED PENIS

FORESKIN

CIRCUMCISED PENIS

HEAD OR GLANS

FORESKIN HAS BEEN REMOVED

Semen

After puberty, sperm are being manufactured in a boy's testicles all the time and stored in the epididymis, a tube attached to each testicle. When a boy is turned on and his penis is erect, his sperm move from his balls into an area at the back of the penis, where they get mixed with a whitish liquid from the prostate gland and seminal vesicles called seminal fluid. Semen is the name we give to the resulting sperm and seminal fluid cocktail that spills out during ejaculation.

Each ejaculation contains about a teaspoon of semen, populated by around 300 million sperm. And it only takes one fast-swimming one to get you pregnant.

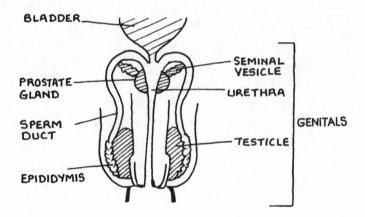

Wet Dreams

We all dream several times a night, and once boys hit puberty, they can get erections when they dream. In the early years, wet dreams, in which a boy ejaculates automatically in his sleep, are common. While wet dreams are more usual in a boy's teens and twenties, they can occur at any age after puberty.

Sometimes they're a reaction to a sexy dream, sometimes not. It might wake him up, or he might only know it's happened by the soggy sheets in the morning. Girls can orgasm in their sleep too.

His Orgasm

When a boy is sexually excited, his penis fills with blood and becomes erect. If his penis is stimulated sufficiently, his body passes through various stages, many similar to a girl's, that will eventually end in an orgasm.

A boy's testicles draw up close to his body, his heart thumps, and he may pant and tense his arms and legs. He might get erect nipples and the sex flush over his chest. At this point a clear liquid, called the pre-ejaculate, leaks out of the penis. Most of this is made in a different part of the body from semen, but it still contains thousands of sperm. Then powerful rhythmic contractions of the boy's penis, anus, and other genital muscles lead to ejaculation, in which semen is forced out of the end of the penis. This is his orgasm.

If a boy is very excited but doesn't come, his testicles might ache (sometimes called "blue balls"). This sensation soon fades and doesn't do any harm—whatever you may hear to the contrary.

CHAPTER TWO
Periods

Periods are a normal and natural part of being a woman. This chapter focuses on how they come about and how to manage them. In it you'll find the lowdown on:

- Your Internal Reproductive System: Womb and Cervix; Fallopian Tubes; Ovaries; Ovulation
- Your Period: First Period; Problem Periods; Pads or Tampons?

YOUR INTERNAL REPRODUCTIVE SYSTEM

It may seem completely weird now, but the main point of puberty is to make you capable of producing babies. And while all the external things we've looked at so far are going on, there are plenty of changes inside you that you won't be aware of.

The outward sign that your reproductive organs are maturing is your period, the process by which your body gets rid of the womb lining each month that wasn't used to nourish a growing baby.

Internally, your reproductive system is made up of your womb and cervix, ovaries, Fallopian tubes, and vagina. Chapter 1 covered the vagina, so this chapter looks at the other organs and how they relate to each other. Here's a diagram to help you work out what's what.

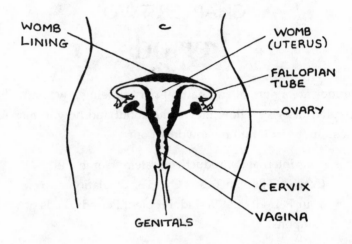

Womb and Cervix

Your womb, or uterus, is a hollow, pear-shaped organ about the size of your fist. Made of muscle, it's capable of expanding massively to hold a baby. The womb tilts forward over your bladder, and we call the lower end the cervix (neck of the womb). The cervix protrudes into the top part of the vagina.

Fallopian Tubes

On either side of and connected to the womb at the top are your Fallopian tubes, which are tubes the thickness of a fine needle. They're each about four inches long, and the outer, open end has fringes that hang over each ovary without touching it.

Ovaries

You have two of these almond-shaped structures, one attached to each side of your womb. They have two main functions:

- to produce eggs;
- to produce the female hormones, estrogen and progesterone, responsible for puberty and controlling your periods (menstrual cycle). (The ovaries also produce small amounts of the male hormone, testosterone.)

You're born with all your eggs, up to 400,000, in your ovaries, although during your lifetime only 300 to 500 of these will mature and be released in the monthly process known as ovulation.

Ovulation

Every month, up to thirty eggs start to ripen, but only one will mature fully and break away from the surface of the ovary. Your ovaries take turns releasing an egg, a process which is called ovulation. This happens roughly fourteen days after the first day of your period. Some girls feel the egg being released as a cramp low in the abdomen or back, and there can be a tiny bit of blood from the vagina.

The cervix secretes different kinds of mucus throughout the month that seep from the vagina, and you'll notice it on toilet paper when you wipe yourself. For a few days after your period, there's not much mucus, and so your vagina will feel a bit dry. Then, for most of the month, the mucus is thick and sticky, like wallpaper paste. Five or six days before ovulation, it's watery. For a couple of days around ovulation, the mucus becomes slippery and stretchy, like egg whites. This "fertile" mucus acts as a transport system for any sperm that may happen along and helps keep it alive on its journey to locate and fertilize your egg.

The released egg, which is the size of a pinhead, floats to the Fallopian tube above it, and the fringes sweep it up inside the tube. Once in the Fallopian tube, wavelike motions draw it down into the womb. If this egg meets a sperm on its journey down the Fallopian tube, the sperm will burrow into it—a process known as fertilization. Unless something interrupts the process, the fertilized egg then nestles into the lining of the womb and starts to grow into a baby. This implantation process is complete about nine days after you've ovulated. If the egg isn't fertilized, as the majority aren't, it breaks up in the womb twenty-four hours after ovulation and comes out along with your period, but you won't notice it.

Over the course of the month, your womb lining has been thickening and getting ready to nourish a baby. If the egg isn't fertilized, the womb lining is shed over several days. Your cervix opens slightly to release the lining. This is your period. Then the cycle beings again.

YOUR PERIOD

Although we talk about periods being every month, in fact the cycle can range from twenty to forty days, with twenty-eight days being the average. A period can last two to eight days, but is generally about five. The fluid you lose is made up of blood, cervical mucus, and secretions from your vagina, although it might appear to be all blood. On average, you lose four to six tablespoons of fluid.

Count day one of your period as the first day you get fresh, red blood. The length of your menstrual cycle is from day one up to, but not including, the first day of your next period.

Lots of girls find their breasts become tender or sore before or during a period and sometimes swell a little. You might also feel bloated. These are due to a build up of fluid in the body at this time, and everything goes back to normal either when your period starts or just after.

First Period

You won't know when your first period is due to begin. However, the age at which you begin menstruating sometimes runs in the family, so if your mother was early or late, you might be too. It used to be thought that the younger you start, the older you'll be when your periods finish (known as menopause), but studies have failed to prove that this is the rule.

The first sign that your periods are on their way is a white discharge from your vagina that you'll notice in your panties up to six months before. This means your hormones are getting into gear.

When your period first starts, it tends to be brownish and there's not much of it. It can take up to eighteen months for your periods to settle into a regular pattern while your hormones are getting the balance right, and early on lots of girls have gaps between periods of between two and six months. During this time, while your periods are settling down, it's common not to release eggs. However, you won't be aware whether you're releasing eggs or not. And it's possible to get pregnant before your period starts, because a girl's first ovulation can occur just before her first period.

Problem Periods

Period Pain

Doctors used to believe that women imagined menstrual pain, but luckily those days are gone. Up to six out of ten girls suffer from it, and a few get such bad pains that they can't go about their usual business. Your hormones cause these cramping pains, and it means your womb is contracting—the muscles are clenching—in a similar way to when your womb is pushing a baby out during birth.

While cramps are the most common kind of period pain, you might get a heavy, dragging feeling in your lower belly and soreness at the bottom of your back or at the top of your inner thighs. Pain is worst during the time of heaviest blood flow.

You might get pain with your very first period, but it's more likely to kick in after six to twelve months. It tends to be worse in the first few years while your body is adjusting your new hormonal levels.

Zapping Period Pain

There's no need to suffer with period pain. Here are some ideas on how to manage it:

- Curl up with a heating pad against your belly or back, depending on where it hurts.
- Take a long, hot bath.
- Massage your stomach and back.
- Exercise gently, even though you may not feel like it. This helps by relaxing your muscles and improving the blood supply to your pelvic region.
- Include dark green, leafy vegetables and nuts in your

daily diet. They contain magnesium and calcium, which nutritional experts say calm the womb muscles.

- You can buy painkillers such as Pamprin or Midol, made especially for period cramps, which work for most people. Your pharmacist can advise you.

- If your pains are really bad, see your doctor, as there are various medications you can get by prescription. Because the contraceptive pill can reduce period pain, your doctor may suggest you take it for this reason even if you're not having sex.

Heavy Periods

If your periods suddenly become heavier and you find you're having to use more pads or tampons than usual, or periods last longer than before, it's generally either due to (a) stress or emotional reasons or (b) a physical problem.

In the first category, a change of routine (for example, moving) or a shock (the death of a relative or friend, or failing exams), can affect your cycle temporarily.

If you haven't changed your routine or been upset about something but the heavy periods continue, it's best to see your doctor so he or she can check your womb and possibly your hormonal balance. Heavy blood loss over time can make you anemic, which needs treatment, normally in the form of iron supplements. (Symptoms of anemia are tiredness, dizziness, headaches, breathlessness, and pale skin in fair girls or grayish skin in dark-skinned girls.) There are prescription drugs that reduce monthly blood loss, and girls who go on the contraceptive pill generally have lighter periods.

Premenstrual Syndrome (PMS)

Another problem caused by those female hormones, PMS, used to be known as premenstrual tension (PMT), but it involves a cluster of symptoms, of which irritability is only one, so we now talk of it as a syndrome.

Researchers have discovered over a hundred PMS symptoms, but here are the most common ones:

- being accident prone
- sore boobs
- irritability and mood swings
- tearfulness
- problems sleeping
- bloated belly
- headaches
- acne
- depression
- feeling faint
- craving sweets
- feeling sick
- tiredness

Up to 90 percent of girls suffer from some form of PMS. You may get both or either period pain and PMS or, if you're lucky, neither! If you have any of the listed symptoms, you can tell they're PMS because they come at the same time every month. Noting down how you feel each day for three months will show you if it's PMS. Then you'll be able to predict when symptoms will occur and will know to take care of yourself on those days. Generally, the symptoms start a few days before your period is due and stop on the first day of bleeding (fresh red blood).

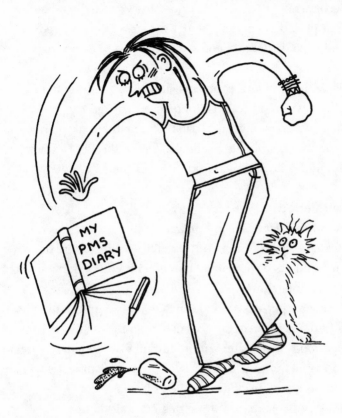

Ways to Reduce Your PMS

* Avoid caffeine, in the form of coffee, soft drinks, and chocolate.
* Eat fewer dairy products; less red meat, salt, and sugar; and more fruit and vegetables.
* Take a good (i.e., not cheap!) multivitamin capsule containing B vitamins, calcium, and magnesium each day. You can buy these from health food stores or pharmacies.
* Exercise at least three times a week for twenty minutes. (Brisk walking will do.)

* Recognize that you'll feel under the weather just before your period. Sometimes that awareness alone can reduce feelings of irritability and make you less likely to snap at people.

* As with all health problems, if you're really suffering, talk to your doctor. Antidepressant drugs can reduce PMS mood swings and irritability, or there are various hormonal treatments available. Again, the Pill can help, although some women find it makes their PMS worse.

Missed Period
If You Haven't Had Sexual Contact

By "sexual contact," I mean any sexual activity where the boy's sperm could have come into contact with your vagina, not just full sexual intercourse.

Once your periods start, it can take up to eighteen months to settle into a regular pattern of one roughly each month. So if your periods have begun within that time and you haven't had sexual contact with a boy, gaps of anywhere from two to six months between periods are quite normal.

Other possible reasons for a missed period are:

• Dieting: losing too much body fat can stop your periods.

• Heavy athletic training: again, because body fat gets too low.

• Stress and other emotional factors: for example, worrying about exams or mourning a death.

• Any change to your routine, such as traveling or starting a new school.

However, it's probably best to have a chat with your doctor or school nurse if you miss more than one period.

If You Have Had Sexual Contact

If you have had sexual intercourse or any sexual contact and your period doesn't arrive, then you may be pregnant—even if you used contraception, because contraception can fail. To find out the facts on contraception, see chapter 10. You'll find information on what to do if you're pregnant in chapter 17.

If you think you might be pregnant, then don't delay: get a pregnancy test done, because the sooner the pregnancy is confirmed, the more choices you have. Tests are sometimes free at family-planning clinics. They're also covered by most medical insurance.

For information on the above and where to find clinics, see "Resources and Contacts" at the back of this book.

If you can afford it, home pregnancy testing kits cost about thirteen dollars from pharmacies, and they're as reliable as the tests done by family-planning clinics. The fact that you get the result within minutes is a big plus.

Pads or Tampons?

There are loads of products on the market to soak up your period flow, but basically it boils down to two forms of protection: internal, provided by tampons, or external, for which you use pads. Here are the advantages and disadvantages of each.

Pads

A trip to the pharmacy or supermarket will show you that there's a mind-boggling array of products to choose from. All have a sticky strip down the middle that you peel the backing from and press onto the crotch of your underwear. It's a good idea to try a few different types to see which suit you best. You can now even buy "string" pads for when you wear thongs, although you'd have to have a very light flow to have enough room on the pad.

Most pads come in normal, super, and nighttime sizes, depending on how much fluid they absorb. Nighttime ones are made to wear while you sleep and are the most absorbent and the longest. If your blood flow is light, or at the start or end of your period when there's less blood, you'll want a thinner pad. These are less likely to show under tight clothes. Thicker, longer, more absorbent pads and ones with wings are best if your flow is heavier, as the two wings, which fold around the crotch, stop blood staining the sides of your underpants. Some manufacturers claim that their ultraslim pads can still hold a lot of fluid.

Changing your pad every two or three hours when your flow is heaviest will make you less likely to stain your panties. Never flush pads down the toilet, no matter what the wrapping says. Sewage systems can't process them, and so they end up clogging the plumbing or washing up on beaches. Put them in the trash or the special disposal units in public toilets. Many pads come individually packaged in colorful wrappings, making them easier to spot in the bottom of your bag.

Advantages of Pads
* Pads can give better protection at night.
* It's obvious when they need changing, so you can't forget.
* You don't have to touch your genital area during a period, as you do with tampons, which some girls prefer.

Disadvantages of Pads

* They can feel bulky and moist.
* They can slip off the adhesive backing and bunch up in your pants.
* Pads are harder to dispose of away from home, as they can be pretty big.
* They can show through tight clothes.
* They can get smelly if not changed often enough.
* You can't go swimming wearing a pad.
* They can feel uncomfortable during some sports (for example, cycling).

Panty Liners

These are short, thin pads that stick to your panties and are useful if you think your period's due, at the beginning and end of a period when there's less blood, and sometimes along with a tampon for extra underwear protection. They're also good for the times of the month when your vaginal secretions are runnier. Panty liners are all roughly the same size, plus there are shapes for use with thongs.

Tampons

Ancient Egyptians used softened papyrus as tampons, but the cottonlike kind that are around today were invented in the 1930s. Like pads, there are lots of brands, but they come in two basic types: with an applicator to help with insertion, and without. Girls have a definite preference for one or the other. Tampax is the most famous with-applicator brand, and OB is the best-known applicator-free brand. All have a string firmly attached that hangs outside of you, which you use to pull the tampon out.

Tampons come in slim, regular, super, and super plus, although you'll find some variation in the names depending on the brand. The size refers to how much blood they can absorb, not the size of your vagina. Having said that, slims are aimed at younger girls, as the tampons are very thin, but if your flow is anything other than minuscule, you'll need one of the more absorbent sizes.

It takes practice to put in a tampon, so if you really want to use them, don't be discouraged if you don't get it right the first time. Insertion instructions are given inside the box.

Advantages of Tampons

* They don't show through your clothes.
* You don't have to worry about odor.
* If it's inserted properly, you can't feel it.
* You can swim and shower with one in.

Disadvantages of Tampons

* You might not know a tampon needs changing until you get a leak.
* They can be hard to get in if your flow is very light, as you need blood for lubrication.
* There is a very small risk of toxic shock syndrome.

Toxic Shock Syndrome (TSS)

This is a rare disease associated with tampon use, and it can be fatal. TSS is caused by bacteria that live harmlessly in the vagina. Under circumstances that aren't clear, sometimes these multiply rapidly, causing blood poisoning. Symptoms come on suddenly and include a high fever, vomiting, dizziness, feeling faint or actually fainting, diarrhea, and a sunburnlike rash. If you have any of these symptoms during a period in which you've used a tampon at some point, or soon after your period, seek medical attention immediately and take the tampon out if you're wearing one.

Reducing Your Risk of TSS

* Change your tampon every four to eight hours. If wearing one to bed, put a fresh one in just before you go to sleep and change it as soon as you wake up.
* Always use the lowest absorbency for your flow. This ensures you'll change it often, as you shouldn't keep the same tampon in for more than eight hours.
* Don't use tampons all through your period. Wear a pad once a day, or at night.
* Make sure you remember to remove the last tampon after your period's finished.

Tampons and Virginity

The fact is, if your hymen is still intact, it nevertheless has one or more openings in it for your period to seep out of. A tampon will slip into one of these openings, although this may enlarge it a little. However, virginity relates to a penis going into a girl's vagina. Therefore there's only one way to lose your virginity, and that's by having sexual intercourse.

CHAPTER THREE

Here's Looking at You

Before we get down to the nitty gritty of sex and relationships, we're going to take a look at bodies, and how you see yourself. In this chapter, you'll find information about:

- Body Image: Your Looks; Your Weight
- Eating Disorders: Anorexia Nervosa; Bulimia Nervosa; Signs of an Eating Disorder; Help for Eating Disorders
- Boobs: What They're Made Of; Big or Small?; Different Sizes; Nipples; Stretch Marks; Checking Your Breasts; Bras; Boob Jobs
- QUIZ: Body Language
- Body Positive: Self-Esteem

BODY IMAGE

So how do you feel about the way you look? There's no denying it's a tough business being a girl in our society. If an alien landed in the United States and tried to learn about the female of the species by watching TV and flicking through a few magazines, he'd assume we're all bone thin, long-legged, flawless beauties who spend all day tossing our shiny hair around.

On billboards and in newspapers and magazines (especially the ever-increasing piles of men's mags), women are often shown half naked in provocative positions. We're big business: in advertising, women's bodies are used to sell everything from perfume to food to vacations.

It doesn't help that many models, actresses, and singers starve themselves and then sculpt their faces and bodies with plastic surgery, leading women and girls to aspire to a "perfection" that doesn't exist in nature. This includes being rail thin with huge boobs, a shape that's virtually impossible to achieve without help because the bigger the boobs, the more fat content they have—so if there's hardly any fat on your body, there sure won't be much in your breasts.

And we even worry about our coloring. Some people find red hair a source of amusement, and many believe that being blond and blue-eyed is still the ideal. This is particularly hard on girls who don't have white skin—although black girls win one round of the beauty battle in that surveys show they're more likely to be content with a curvier figure. The good news is that as our society becomes more multicultural, the standards of beauty are slowly changing to include role models from every race.

Your Looks

One thing's for sure: there's a huge range of body shapes and sizes, facial features, hair types, and all the other parts and pieces that make up our overall appearance. You may be tall, short, or in between, with a nose that's large, small, turned up or flat. Lips range from full to thin, and often the bottom lip is plumper than the top one. Face shapes come in round, heart shaped, long, or squareish, framed by hair that can be poker straight, wild and frizzy, or gently waving. The point is that we're all different, all unique, but few girls are totally happy with how they look, even those who fit into whatever image the media is currently peddling. According to a recent survey in a teen magazine, nine out of ten readers are unhappy with their looks. And this is such a shame, because however much you dislike parts of yourself and think that no one will ever like you because of your butt/thighs/breasts, etc., it's really not true.

However you look, the best thing you can do for yourself is learn to accept what you've got, and this chapter is about helping you to do this. "Beauty is in the eye of the beholder" may be a cliché, but it's absolutely true that what turns one person off is the answer to another's wildest dreams. Just look around you at couples of all ages and you'll see an enormous variation in what people find attractive.

Your Weight

Of course, the constant parade of super-skinny women with every tiny blemish airbrushed out makes most of us, even those who are slim, feel fat and inadequate. The diet industry (books, weight-loss clubs, diet foods, supplements, videos, and the like) is big business and is worth many millions of dollars a year. But think about it: if it were that easy to shed the pounds and keep them off, then why would people keep going back to weight-loss clubs and why would there be a new diet craze on the market every few months?

Now I'm going to share a secret with you that the diet industry doesn't want you to know: DIETS DON'T WORK LONG TERM. Yeah, yeah, yeah, you've heard it all before, but listen up for a minute. Lots of studies show that yes, people lose weight initially, but the vast majority put all that lost weight back on within a year. This happens for two reasons. First, when you deprive your body of fuel in the form of calories, you quickly lose fluids, which shows up as weight loss when you step on the scale. Next, your body starts burning your lean tissue (muscle) for energy if you're not using it (i.e., exercising), not your fat, which means you start to lose muscle. Second, as time passes, the dieter gets tired of eating a limited range of foods and is back on their normal diet. Result: the weight soon goes back on—as fat.

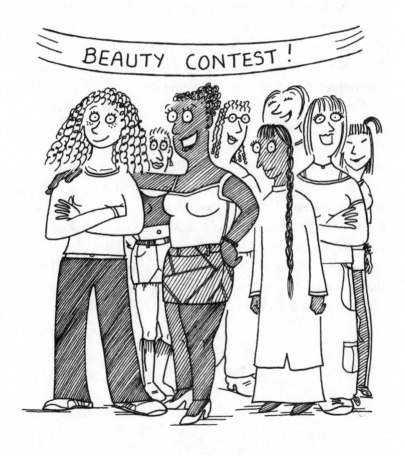

Dieting leaves you with more fat and less muscle than before you started. So, feeling like porky failures, what do many of us do next? You've guessed it: we look for another "miracle" diet!

It's much better for your body to think in terms of getting toned and healthy rather than getting skinny, and long-term healthy eating plus exercise in moderation are the keys to this. Muscle burns more calories than fat, even when you're asleep, and you can only build muscle from exercising. There are loads of sports to choose from, and playing or exercising with friends makes it more fun, plus you can motivate each other. For example, walking is easy to fit into your life, and it's free. Build up to thirty minutes a day three or four times a week. Swimming is another good, all-round exercise.

Depriving yourself totally of foods you love but that may not be good for you is a sure way to get yourself craving them, so think of it this way: some nutritionists suggest that as long as 80 percent of what you eat is healthy—low in salt, sugar, and fat; fish, chicken, and lean meat; fresh fruit and veggies; whole-grain bread, cereals, rice, and pasta; and low-fat dairy foods—then you can indulge in small portions of the foods you enjoy for the other 20 percent of your food intake.

Getting healthy is about making changes to your lifestyle that you can stick to, and doing this gradually. There are no quick fixes, whatever the latest celeb endorsements say.

EATING DISORDERS

I've had girls write to me asking how they can get anorexia, because they're so desperate to be thin. But eating disorders are no joke. According to the National Eating Disorders Association (NEDA), they're most common among young women aged fifteen to twenty-five. Up to one of every hundred young women suffers from anorexia, and up to three in every hundred are bulimic. Some people might have a mixture of anorexia and bulimia.

A person is considered to have an eating disorder if they're obsessed with food, eating, and/or their weight and shape. Often they're also deeply distressed about things in their life that aren't related to dieting and food. They might feel depressed and unhappy about themselves and use food as a way of coping with these feelings. In general, the person feels they have little control over their life, and the only thing they can control is what they eat. Low self-esteem is thought to be at the root of all eating disorders.

The link between dieting and eating disorders is complex, but some experts believe that for girls who develop an eating disorder, dieting is a symptom that they're at risk of using food to manage their psychological problems rather than the cause of the illness.

Anorexia Nervosa

In its most common form, girls with anorexia are terrified of gaining weight and will insist on remaining underweight. Even when at a very low weight, they'll still see themselves as being fat. Their periods often stop and their hair may start to fall out.

They might pretend they've eaten meals and exercise excessively to keep the weight off.

There are also people who eat normal amounts, start an exercise program to get fit, and then slide into overexercising without realizing it and wind up needing help. Anorexia has one of the highest death rates of any psychiatric condition, with between five and twenty out of every hundred sufferers dying each year from the effects of starvation and low body weight, says the NEDA.

Bulimia Nervosa

At its most extreme, bulimia sufferers have comfort-eating binges during which they'll eat abnormally large quantities of food, feeling out of control of what they eat during the binge. Then, to keep from putting on weight, they might make themselves vomit, use laxatives, diet strictly, or exercise excessively. Other sufferers may eat normal meals, but use vomiting, laxatives, or loads of exercise to control their weight. Like anorexics, people with bulimia also judge themselves harshly on the way they look.

Signs of an Eating Disorder

If you answer yes to any of the following questions, you may have an eating disorder:

- Do you feel fat even though people tell you how thin you are?
- Do you think about food all the time?
- Do you feel fear, guilt, anger, or shame when faced with food?
- Do you get anxious if you can't exercise to burn off calories?

- Do you worry about your weight, figure, and how much you eat all the time?
- Have your periods become irregular or stopped completely?
- Are other people talking about the way you eat?
- Do you lie about what you eat?
- When you eat, are you afraid you won't be able to stop?
- Do you vomit or take laxatives to control your weight?
- Do you feel alone with your struggle with food and your weight?
- Do you feel you'd be happier, more acceptable, and more successful if you lost weight?
- Do you feel depressed about yourself and use food to cope with these feelings?

Adapted from the ANRED (Anorexia Nervosa and Related Eating Disorders, Inc.) Web site at http://www.anred.com.

Help for Eating Disorders

If you think you might suffer from an eating disorder, the first step to recovery is admitting to yourself that you have a problem. Sufferers often deny they're ill and may conduct their food rituals (for example, bingeing, vomiting, and stockpiling food) in secret. You might feel guilty or ashamed, but the eating disorder is a sign that you need help in coping with other areas of your life. Your doctor can put you in touch with helpful services. You'll find more suggestions in the "Resources and Contacts" section of this book.

BOOBS

Love 'em or hate 'em, we've all got a pair under our sweaters. And the grass is always greener in another girl's bra, so to speak. If you're on the small side, you dream of having grapefruits to show off in a tight tee. If you're busty, you're desperate for them to shrink so boys will look you in the eye rather than stare at your chest. Who'd have thought two mounds of flesh could cause so much heartache?

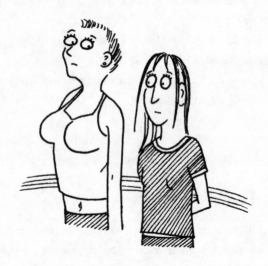

What They're Made Of

For many girls, breast development at about ten or eleven or thereabouts, is the first sign that puberty's beginning. Your breasts reach their full adult size when you're eighteen or nineteen, give or take a year. They're made of fatty tissue, with small milk-producing glands connected to the nipple. While we all have a similar number of glands, some girls have more fat there than others, which accounts for the variations in size. The nipple is surrounded by a circular area of skin called the areola. This has oil glands on it, which you'll notice as small bumps. The nipple and areola range in color from pale pink to dark brown, depending on your skin color.

Big or Small?

Some girls with small boobs complain of feeling less feminine. And if you're big up top, some boys think you're promiscuous and it can seem like they're not interested in anything else about you. But whatever their size, breasts are all capable of giving sexual pleasure to you and your partner, so try and be proud of what you've got. In the same way that you and your friends don't all like the same boy, boys love boobs and bodies in all shapes and sizes, regardless of the latest look. And, believe it or not, plenty choose a girlfriend for her personality and sense of fun and don't give a monkey's butt about what's going on in her bra!

Different Sizes

If you split a photo of your face down the middle and matched each half up with its mirror image, you'd see that the two sides of your face are pretty different. In fact, the right and left sides of our entire body are slightly asymmetrical, and the same goes for your boobs. This is particularly true while they're growing, because each boob might grow at a different rate. They usually catch up, although one will often remain a bit bigger than the other.

When you're fully grown, you might find the difference between them is very marked. This is totally normal, and most girls learn to live with it. But if it bothers you, try padding in one bra cup.

For girls who are very miserable about having uneven breasts, it's possible either to have the larger one reduced or the smaller one enlarged with cosmetic surgery (see "Boob Jobs" on pages 48–50). Medical insurance won't pay for this unless a psychiatrist recommended it be done because the unevenness was causing you extreme mental distress, which is very rare!

Nipples

Your nipples may stick out, lie flat, or be inverted and look like slits. Or you might have just one that's inverted. Sometimes, as your boobs continue to grow, the nipple gets pushed outward. But if yours stay in, remember that it's perfectly normal and you'll still be able to breast-feed a baby if you want to in later life.

If you're cold, sexually excited, nervous, or something rubs against them, nipples can become erect and pop out.

Stretch Marks

It's common to get stretch marks on your breasts, because sometimes they grow so fast inside that your skin hasn't had enough time to grow, so it stretches instead. These lines can look alarming at first, but they do fade and become less obvious. Stretch marks on fair skins turn a silvery color, while darker-skinned girls find theirs end up a little paler than the surrounding skin.

Checking Your Breasts

Although breast cancer is rare in teenagers, it's a good idea to get into the habit of checking your boobs each month. That way you get to know what's normal for you and are in a better position to notice any changes.

A few days after your period has ended is a good time, as the breast tissue will be less tender. First, take off your bra and look in the mirror with your hands raised over your head. You're looking for any changes in boob shape or in the color and texture of the skin and nipples or a discharge from the nipples.

Next, lie down with one hand behind your head and, using the flat surface of the three middle fingers (not your fingertips) of your left hand, think of your right breast as the face of a clock. Using medium pressure, move your fingers in small circles from the twelve o' clock position under the collarbone all the way around. Then do the same farther in around your nipple. Check around your armpit as well, then repeat with the other hand on your left breast. This can also be done in the shower with soapy fingers, but remember to raise the arm above your head on the side you're checking.

While breast cancer is uncommon in teenagers, benign (non-cancerous) lumps in the breasts crop up due to a sensitivity to female hormones, plus everyone has bumpy areas that are unique to them. It's important to find out what's usual for you and see your doctor if anything worries you. If you're nervous about talking to your doctor, see chapter 13.

Many girls find the thought of touching or examining their breasts a bit weird. Others are scared to do it in case they find something worrysome. But you and your boobs are going to be together for a while, so isn't it time you were properly introduced?

Bras

There's a huge array of bras on the market to help you look bigger, smaller, have more cleavage, to wear during sports, with halter tops, with T-shirts, etc. But whatever kind you like, the vital thing is that you wear the right size—and most girls don't. Sounds obvious, but if your bra has loose areas it's too big, and if flesh bulges over the cups, it's too small.

Many girls just guess and snatch the first bra they like the look of off the rack, which is a mistake. There are no muscles in your boobs—they're held up by suspensory ligaments. If you don't wear a bra, or wear one that's not supporting you properly, these stretch and your breasts will start to droop, particularly if they're heavy. Once this has happened, nothing short of surgery will correct it, so it makes sense to find out your size.

The best way to do this is to get measured by a professional and talk with that person about what you want from a bra. You'll need to be remeasured if you gain or lose weight. Any department store that sells bras will have someone who can measure you. And try not to worry about what they'll think of your chest. They've seen every possible size and shape before!

Boob Jobs

Breast Enlargement
We seem to have a national obsession with plastic surgery. In particular, magazines and newspapers devote much space to speculating about which female celebs have had boob jobs. So what *is* a boob job?

Generally, people are talking about breast enlargement. This is where the surgeon makes a slit under each breast (or it can be under the arm or around the nipple) and pushes a bag inside containing either a salt–water solution or silicone gel to increase the size of the breasts.

False breasts feel firmer than real breasts and stick up when you're lying down, rather than flop to the sides like naturally large boobs. Most medical insurance plans do not cover enlargements. So if you're unhappy with small boobs you'll have to pay out of pocket to have them done, and no reputable surgeon would operate on a girl until her breasts had reached their full adult size. You can usually still breast-feed after a boob enhancement.

When we read in a magazine that so-and-so has had her cup size surgically boosted, there's little mention of the fact that, like all operations, breast enlargement carries health risks and recovery can be painful. And while plenty of women's breast implants are fine, there are problems associated with them, including infections around the implants, numb nipples, the entire implant hardening, or the contents of the bag inside the breast leaking. A few women believe their implants have brought on an arthritis-like condition in their joints.

The fact is, cosmetic surgery is never the answer to your problems, however seductive the idea might seem. Many people who have one area operated on feel better for a while, but then shift their focus to another body part and obsess about that. Far better to accept what nature gave you and work on improving your overall confidence. Remember, something can only make you unhappy if you go over it repeatedly in your mind. Why not put your mental energy into something more worthwhile?

Breast Reduction

This is a major operation that's sometimes paid for by insurance, but, again, not until a girl's breasts are fully developed. It's generally done on older women who've had children and whose breasts have drooped a lot. Backache, neck pain, and dents in your shoulders from your bra having to support very heavy breasts, plus boobs so big that your movement is restricted are the other reasons women get this done. In other words, it's normally done for health reasons rather than just to look better.

Breast reduction involves reducing the size of the breast surgically and then repositioning the nipple. You can lose nipple sensation and some women can't breast-feed afterward. Noticeable scars are usual.

QUIZ: BODY LANGUAGE

What does your attitude toward your body say about you? Try this quiz to check out how you see yourself. At the end, you'll find tips on how to feel great whatever your size and shape.

Answer the following questions by circling the number in the Yes or No columns. Then add up the numbers to see which type you are.

	YES	NO
1. Are you happy with your body generally?	3	0
2. Would you consider cosmetic surgery if it were free?	0	1
3. Would you like a makeover?	1	2
4. Do you wish you had more confidence?	1	3
5. Do your friends pay you compliments?	1	0

6.	Can you find lots of styles that suit you in stores?	3	1
7.	Would you like to change your hair color?	1	2
8.	Are you jealous of other girls' looks?	0	2
9.	Are you often on a diet?	1	2
10.	Do you think your life would be better if you looked different?	0	3
11.	Do you spend a lot on beauty and hair products?	1	2
12.	Do you ever avoid looking in mirrors?	0	1
13.	Do you think boys might find you attractive?	2	0
14.	Is there something you'd like to change about your looks?	1	2
15.	Are you on a diet now?	1	3
16.	Do you usually wear black rather than bright colors?	0	2
17.	Are you comfortable in a swimsuit?	3	0
18.	Do you dress in the latest fashions?	2	1
19.	Are you confident with boys?	3	0
20.	Do people say you're fun?	3	0
21.	Do you get lots of male attention?	3	0
22.	Do you always put makeup on before you go out?	1	2
23.	Do you go shopping every weekend?	1	2
24.	Would you say you're fat?	0	2
25.	Do you hide any part of your body?	1	2

1–14 POINTS: SELF-CONSCIOUS

You have very low self-esteem and a poor body image. There's not much you like about yourself, and you think your main problem is your body. Whether you think you're too fat, too skinny, have mousy hair or a big nose, you're so self-conscious that you scuttle away whenever someone tries to talk to you. But real happiness comes from within, and the more you like yourself for being you, the more attractive you'll become to everyone else. Think about all those celebs that are, and let's be frank about this, pretty ugly, but because they carry themselves with confidence they ooze charisma and are practically beating off potential partners with a stick. So forget that nose or boob job, liposuction or miracle diet, and start learning to like yourself. You'll soon see a change in how you feel.

15–27 POINTS: SHY

The good news is that you don't have a big problem with self-image. You quite like who you are and know you have lots to offer. The bad news is that you're so reserved that you never let anyone see the real you. You have good friends and are well liked, even though you might not believe that. You need to have more confidence in yourself. The happier and more sure of yourself you seem, the more attractive you'll be. And that's the key: some people spend thousands of dollars on cosmetic surgery, fancy diets, or designer clothes, but if they're not confident, they won't shine. So believe in yourself, baby!

28–39 POINTS: SATISFIED

This is probably the category most girls fall into. You're a happy-go-lucky person who makes an effort to look good. You love clothes and know all the tricks to minimize the body parts that bother you, like wearing black to flatter wider hips. There are quite a few things you don't like about the way you look, and you worry about them a bit too much. You're doing OK, but keep an eye out to make sure you don't slide into obsessing about one particular feature. If that happens, take time to chill out and make a list of everything that's good about your life.

40+ POINTS: SET

Congratulations, Ms. Well Balanced! You're happy with who you are, inside and out. People are drawn to you like a magnet because you exude confidence, sex appeal, and happiness. You have bad days, but you can draw on your inner confidence to get you through them. You may not have a supermodel body, but you don't give a damn because you like who you are. Others can learn a lot from you. You have your own sense of style and don't care what the latest fashion is, because whatever you wear, you can carry it off. Way to go, girl!

BODY POSITIVE

From the quiz, you'll have an idea whether you need to make changes to what's going on in your head. So read on if you want to feel better (or *even* better!) about yourself.

Self-Esteem

What exactly is this thing called self-esteem that everyone is always going on about? In a nutshell, if you have high self-esteem, you appreciate and accept yourself whatever your achievements and whatever you look like. You accept the negative aspects of your personality as well as the positive ones.

People with low self-esteem don't value themselves and don't feel worthy of good things. They end up treating themselves and others badly, often without meaning to. Having said that, the issue of self-esteem isn't simply that black and white. We all have bad days and good days, but you may find you fall more into one category than the other.

Boosting Your Self-Esteem

It's easy to fall into the trap of believing you'd feel better if you could change your looks or body. Not true. It's the other way around: changing the way you think will help you feel better about how you look. Your thoughts trigger feelings, and feelings lead to behavior. For example, **thought:** *"I'm so fat, no one will ever like me"* might lead to **feeling:** misery, leading to **behavior:** refusing a night out with the girls and slumping on the sofa with a tub of Häagen-Dazs instead.

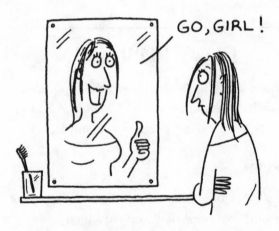

BUILDING SELF-ESTEEM

It might sound corny, but by repeating positive phrases to yourself over and over, eventually they'll sink into your unconscious mind and change the beliefs you have about yourself. So pick three or four phrases to repeat whenever you have time, and jot them down. State what you want, rather than what you don't want, and avoid judgmental words like *fat*, *ugly*, and *horrible*. For example, "I am worthy of love" rather than, "I don't want people to hate me."

When negative thoughts creep into your head, rather than dwelling on them and getting more and more miserable, say, out loud or in your head, "Stop!" Then substitute one of your positive phrases and repeat it over and over. Use these positive thoughts, known as *affirmations*, in any area you want to improve. You can have relationship affirmations, exam affirmations, or any kind you like! Changing how you feel about yourself will make people treat you differently. Try the following:

- I feel happier each day.
- I'm learning to accept my body the way it is.
- I feel calm and relaxed.
- People love to be around me.
- I love and accept myself.

More Tips on Feeling Good

* Work out what you're good at, do more of it, and praise yourself regularly.
* If you want something, ask for it! Giving makes others feel good, and daring to ask makes you feel worthy of getting things you want. Don't be hesitant, and use the word *I*. For example, instead of saying, "Might it be possible for me to . . . ?" say, "I would like . . ." or "I need . . ."
* Be kind to yourself and give yourself treats.
* Talk to friends you trust about things you find hard to deal with.

* Allow yourself to express difficult feelings, such as shame and embarrassment, rather than pretending to be perfect. No one is!
* Separate your behavior from yourself. If you do something silly, it doesn't make you a bad person or mean that *you're* silly.
* Don't put yourself or others down.
* Give more compliments, and accept with thanks those that you're given.
* Concentrate on what you get right rather than on mistakes.

Your self-esteem-boosting program won't work overnight, but if you keep at it, you'll see improvements sooner than you think.

CHAPTER FOUR
Body Q & A

This chapter covers these ten common questions about bodies:

- Do I smell fishy?
- Why do my genitals itch?
- What's a Pap smear?
- How can I get rid of my cellulite?
- Have I lost my tampon?
- Why does my tampon stick out?
- How can I make my boobs bigger?
- Is this an extra breast?
- Should I shave my hairy tummy and face?
- What can I do to lose weight?

Do I smell fishy?

My brother's friends keep joking about girls smelling "fishy." I'm not sure what they're talking about, but how can I make sure I don't smell fishy too?

The boys are referring to the odor of a girl's genital area. Boys know girls worry about how they smell, and that such an insult is extremely hurtful and bound to cause a reaction, which is the object of all bullying and teasing. You'd have to get very close to a girl to know how her genitals smelled, so the insults rarely have any basis in reality. The truth is, boys actually find the scent of a girl's clean genitals exciting. Having said that, while vaginal secretions have only a mild smell, because there are sweat glands in your genital area and you pee from down there, if a girl doesn't wash regularly the combination can result in a slightly fishy odor. A daily wash with unperfumed soap so as not to disturb your vagina's chemical balance is all you need to keep unwanted odors at bay. If you notice an offensive smell, unusual discharge, or itching, see your doctor, as you might have an infection.

Why do my genitals itch?

Recently my vagina started to feel sore and itchy. I haven't done anything sexual with my boyfriend, but could I somehow have caught a sexually transmitted disease?

It sounds like you've got a yeast infection. Besides a sore, itchy vagina, there can also be a vaginal discharge a bit like cottage cheese that smells yeasty, and it may hurt to pee. A yeast infection is caused by an organism that usually lives harmlessly in your vagina and bottom. You can get this without ever having had sex with someone if, for example, you're run down or have been taking antibiotics, which can change your body's chemical balance and allow the bug to spread. Other triggers include being on the Pill, irritation from perfumed bubble bath or soaps, or wearing tight pants or synthetic panties, which cause the kind of warm conditions the yeast thrives on. A yeast infection can also be caught easily during sex. For a proper diagnosis and treatment, see your doctor. Then if the symptoms reoccur, you can treat yourself with a cream called Monistat, available from pharmacies. You should never have sex if you have an infection, and when you're better, always use condoms to protect against pregnancy and new infections. For more on yeast infections, see chapter 11.

What's a Pap smear?

I recently had sex for the first time, and my friends said I need to have a smear. What is it and does it hurt?

You should have your first Pap test done by the time you're twenty-one, or within three years of your first sexual experience. A doctor or nurse slips a metal speculum into your vagina, which widens it slightly so they can see your cervix (neck of your womb). Next, he or she scrapes a few cells from the cervix with a wooden spatula, which looks like a popsicle stick. The cells are put on a slide that's sent off to a lab to be checked for early changes in the cells that could lead to cervical cancer if not treated. Cervical cancer won't develop if these early changes are spotted and dealt with. Smears aren't usually done on young women under twenty-one unless they're sexually active because their bodies are still developing (which can sometimes lead to normal cells being mistaken for abnormal ones) and because cervical cancer is rare in younger women. Smears are done at your gynecologist's office or at a family-planning clinic. Having a smear can be embarrassing, but it usually doesn't hurt and only takes a few minutes. You can arrange to have it done by a female doctor if you prefer.

How can I get rid of my cellulite?

I'm fairly thin, but I've started to notice cellulite on my bottom and thighs. It upsets me so much I can't look in the mirror. How can I get rid of it?

Cellulite is a dimpling of the fleshier areas of the body caused by female hormones, and it's usually most noticeable on the bottom and thighs. Loads of girls have it to some degree. Exercising regularly, drinking lots of water, and eating plenty of fruit and veggies may help. Some people also find that rubbing vitamin E cream into the affected areas improves the look of the skin, but beware: despite the miracle claims of various products, you'll probably just have to learn to live with it. Your skin probably looks worse to you because that's what you're focusing on when you look at your body, but I bet other people aren't that conscious of it.

Have I lost my tampon?

I don't remember taking my tampon out after the end of my period and I'm worried it's gotten lost inside me. I can't see a string—what on earth's happened to it?

Don't worry—it can't get lost because there's nowhere for it to go. At the top of your vagina is your cervix, which has a tiny hole in it the thickness of a straw, and no tampon can get through there. To check if the tampon's still in, sit on the toilet and insert a finger into your vagina. If the tampon's there, you should be able to slide it out. If it's gone, you'll touch your cervix, which feels like the tip of your nose with a dimple in it. But if you're still not sure, get your doctor to take a look as soon as possible. If you leave a tampon inside your body for more than eight hours, you could develop an infection. Tampons that have been left in a long time can very occasionally cause a serious illness called toxic shock syndrome (see pages 34–35), so don't ignore it.

Why does my tampon stick out?

I've recently changed from pads to tampons but I don't think I'm putting them in correctly because some of the tampon sticks out and this hurts. What am I doing wrong?

First of all, have a good look at the instructions enclosed in the box. You probably need to push the tampon in farther. You might find that tampons with applicators are easiest while you're getting used to them. Also, make sure it's at a heavier point in your period, as the blood will act as a lubricant to help the tampon slide in. You aim the tampon toward the bottom of your back, not straight up, and push the cardboard or plastic tube into your vagina until your fingers come into contact with the outside of your body. Then slowly push the smaller tube all the way into the larger one. When you remove both tubes, the tampon should be inside you with only the removal string showing. There's a ring of muscle at the entrance of your vagina, and the tampon should sit above this. If the tampon's in properly, you won't be able to feel it. Relax if you can, because if you're tense, these muscles tighten, which may make insertion hurt and prevent you from being able to get the tampon in.

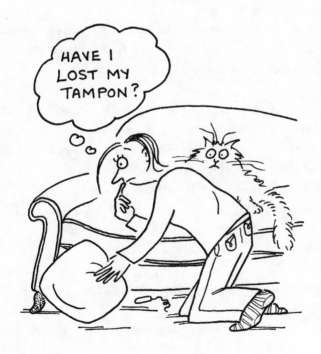

How can I make my boobs bigger?

I'm a 32A bra size and I'm desperate for bigger breasts. I'd do anything—what can you suggest? I'm fifteen.

Despite what the advertisements say, there is absolutely no cream, gadget, or pill that will make boobs larger. Breasts contain no muscles, so exercising won't make any difference either. Often your breasts don't reach their full adult size until your late teens, so there's a fair chance they'll increase in size on their own. Your best bet is to learn to love what you've got, and if you really want a boost, check out push-up and padded bras. Loads of boys are into small, pert boobs!

Is this an extra breast?

I'm fourteen and I have this weird brown lump below one of my boobs, which looks like a pimple, or even a nipple. Both my boobs look normal apart from that. I'm so worried—is it breast cancer?

It sounds like you're describing an extra nipple, known as a "supernumerary" nipple, and they're not uncommon. These tend to be underneath one of your breasts and look a bit like a mole. But don't worry—it's very rare for it to swell like a normal boob, so it's unlikely to become any more noticeable. Breast cancer is very rare in your age group, but it's a good idea to get any odd bumps or lumps checked by your doctor just to be safe, so please make an appointment.

Should I shave my hairy tummy and face?

I want to wear short tops, but I've got dark hairs on my stomach and I'm too embarrassed. I've also got a faint mustache that my friends laugh at. Should I shave this hair off?

It's perfectly normal to have hair on your stomach and top lip. Shaving body hair, apart from legs and armpits, isn't a great idea because you'll get stubble. Bleaching is popular for stomachs and lips, as that makes the hair less noticeable. There's a cream bleach called Jolēn that you could try. If you'd prefer to get rid of it, how about waxing? It can be painful at first, but it gets easier the more you do it. Nair makes a range of waxing products, including mini-strips especially for your face and other delicate areas, such as the bikini line (the hairs visible outside your panty edges). Waxing pulls hair out at the roots, so regrowth is much slower than with shaving or depilatory (hair-removing) creams. Plus the brand-new hairs that grow from the root have tapered tips, so regrowth after waxing is finer than with shaving and depilatory creams, where the hair is sliced off at the skin's surface.

What can I do to lose weight?

I know people say you shouldn't diet, but I feel so chunky that I really need to do something, as it really gets me down. I don't think I can live without chocolate totally, though. What can I do?

Your body changes in your teens, and that means gaining fat and muscle. Your body needs to do this in order to mature. For example, you have to reach a certain weight before your period starts. Also, your hips widen and you develop fat on your bottom and thighs. This new womanly shape can be a bit of a shock, but in time you'll not only get used to it, you might even find you like your new curves! Although flicking through magazines might lead you to believe the world is pop- ulated by super-skinny size-six waifs, it's not true. The average woman in the United States is a size twelve. It's hard to be objective about our own bodies, and many of us see ourselves as fatter than we actually are. But all of us need to exercise to maintain our fitness, so look for an activity that you can do regularly to tone your figure, such as cycling, brisk walking, or Roller blading. Rather than dieting, which is bad for you, think in terms of changing your eating habits for the sake of your health. Choose plenty of fresh fruit and veggies, lean meat, and whole grain bread and pasta. And you can have your chocolate, french fries, and potato chips, but as occasional treats rather than every day. If you need snacks between meals, go for fruit, nuts, and yogurt.

PART TWO

Emotions and You

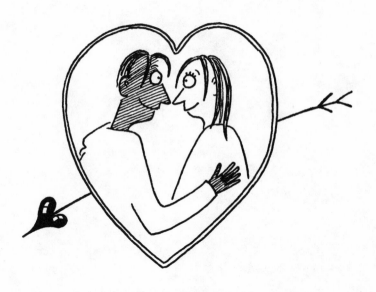

CHAPTER FIVE
The Dating Game

OK. You've read about your body and his body, and thought about how you see yourself. This next section is all about the role your emotions play in sex and relationships.

This chapter looks at attraction, first dates, and actually being in a relationship in the following order:

- Attraction: What's Attraction?; Choosing a Partner; Your Attraction Factor; Do You Like Him?; Does He Like You?
- QUIZ: Boy Gauge—What's He After?
- Dating: Asking Him Out; How to Have a Great Date; Are You Ready to Date?
- Having a Boyfriend: Pairing Up; Is It Love?; Fights; Jealousy; Two-Timing; Breaking Up; Should I Get Back with Him?

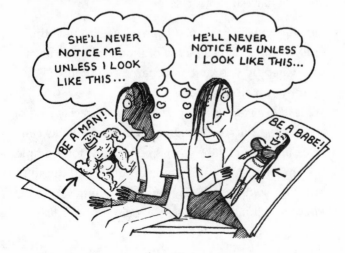

ATTRACTION

What's Attraction?

A strange business, that's what. Although we often think of it in terms of someone's looks or personality, there's a whole lot more to it, including how a person smells (known as *pheromones*, someone's own personal scent), how they treat you, and their body language. For example, you might be chatting to an average-looking dude whose idea of wit doesn't exactly have you rolling in the aisles. Then he moves in for a kiss and *wham!* Before you know it, your knees are shaking, your head's spinning, and you're desperate to see him again!

Although we don't know exactly what sexual chemistry is, psychologists have gathered some evidence on why people get together.

Choosing a Partner

Note that the points in italics are what *tend* to happen in relationships, not hard-and-fast rules.

- *Looks are important for first impressions.* But note this is only *initially*. There's plenty of time for him to be captivated by your wit and charm, so if you've got your eye on an über-babe, go for it!
- *We tend to end up with people of a similar level of physical attractiveness to ourselves.* But one person's looks can be balanced out by the other's personality; for example, the boy may stop traffic while his girlfriend doesn't, but she's so funny all his friends envy him.
- *Pleasant, warm people are seen as more attractive than*

cold, distant ones. However, we all know cool guys and ice maidens with their own fan clubs. Their attraction is probably based on the idea that you might be the one person who can thaw them out. Watch out, though—cool and aloof equals hurtful if they can't relate to other people.

- *Relationships that last are usually between people who share values and attitudes on the important stuff.* Often that means their families behave in similar ways, even if they have different religious or cultural backgrounds. For example, if your family is loving and affectionate toward you, it's likely that you'll feel most comfortable with an affectionate guy.

Your Attraction Factor

I'm so ugly compared to my friends and I can never think what to say to boys. Everyone I know has a boyfriend but me, and I'm terrified I'll never get one. Please help.

Jessica, 16

The big myth about sex appeal is that only the gorgeous, busty, skinny girls get and keep the decent boys. This is baloney. Everyone is attractive to someone. The sad thing about Jessica is that she's so convinced she has nothing to offer a boy that I bet her body language practically screams at them to keep away. If you keep your head down, sit slumped in a chair, drape your hair across your face, and start mumbling whenever a boy speaks to you, or, worse still, run away, then that's not attractive and it will turn boys off.

So how *do* you attract boys? Although I've mentioned body language, drawing people to you isn't about twirling your hair flirtatiously, peering up through your bangs in a girlie manner, shoving your cleavage in boys' faces, or pouting till your lips ache. Yes, some girls do these things and get the guys, but if it doesn't come naturally to you, you'll end up feeling like an idiot rather than a sexpot.

But there are secrets to getting dates. Here they are:

Be Friendly, Interested in the Other Person, and Fun

Instead of pretending you're invisible, or rambling on about your ingrown toenail and mom's hysterectomy, oblivious to whether your chosen guy has fallen into a coma with boredom, ask him about himself. Look him in the eye, listen carefully to his answers, and comment on them. And don't forget to smile!

I'm not saying that you should never talk about the less positive aspects of your life to boys, but be careful. Too much negativity early on puts a boy off and marks you out as a whiner, so wait until you know him better.

Be Yourself

You've heard this one before. But what does it mean? It means that being the way you are with your best friend—chilled, humorous, unselfconscious—is the best way to act around boys. True, this isn't easy at first, but the more boys you talk to, the less scary they'll become as a species, and you'll slowly learn to relax around them. Practice makes perfect, so speak to as many people as you can. As well as getting asked out, you'll make lots of new friends of both sexes!

Make the Most of Yourself

Seeing that a girl's done her best with what God gave her is attractive, whereas looking like you don't care about yourself is a major turnoff. A girl who's made an effort to wash her hair, dress in something not stained with her lunch, and banish dog breath by way of her toothbrush is always going to score points over the slob with scuffed shoes and sweat-stained armpits. Well-cut hair is easier to style, and if you're short on cash, loads of hairdressers will cut your hair cheaply on model days, when their students need someone to practice on (well-supervised, of course). And you can flip through your magazines for ideas on what to wear.

We're brainwashed into thinking we can't look good unless we're experts with the eye-shadow and lip-gloss brushes, but lots of girls find that going makeup free expresses their personality better. However, if you really want to wear makeup and aren't sure what will suit you, get a free makeover at a department store beauty counter.

Do You Like Him?

Sometimes, it's obvious you like someone. Your heart flips like a fish when he's near, you're dying to grab him, and you want to be with him all the time. That's physical attraction, and it hits you like a thunderbolt. But attraction can also be more mental: he's interesting, he makes you giggle, and you enjoy his company. Then it's a lot less clear how we feel. Ideally, you get the physical and mental vibes from the same boy, but it's when you're in the second situation that you find yourself thinking, "Yes, but do I want to go out with him?"

Thing is, the physical thunderbolt thing feels fantastic, but it may not last, and that's when you need the mental aspect as well. The only way to find out if there's mileage in the relationship is to spend more time with the guy. "Time will tell" may be a cliché, but it's certainly true with relationships.

Does He Like You?

If I had a dollar for every letter I've gotten asking how you can tell whether a boy likes you, I'd be writing this from my private jet as I zoom off to my very own Spanish island. Truth is, it's not that hard to work out if a boy has some interest in you. What is tricky, and takes time (there it is again) to discover, is whether they want you

1. as a friend,
2. for kissing,
3. for sex and nothing else, or
4. as a girlfriend.

To really baffle you, a boy might start out wanting one of the first three and then decide you're girlfriend material. Or he might think he wants to go out with you and later change his mind to 1, 2, or 3. But stay with me, because there are clues to what's going on.

Just remember that relationships aren't black and white, however much we'd like them to be. This quick quiz will give you some idea what he's up to, but if in doubt, do more research (i.e., spend more time with him).

QUIZ: BOY GAUGE— WHAT'S HE AFTER?

With a particular boy in mind, decide which of the three situations best completes each question, then circle the color at the end of the line.

1. PHYSICAL

Does he

find excuses to touch your private areas, e.g., boobs and butt?	**Red**
stand or sit comfortably close to you?	**Pink**
stand or sit farther away than you'd like?	**Blue**

2. OTHER PEOPLE

Does he

speak to you in a low voice to keep others from joining in?	**Pink**
bring others into your conversation?	**Blue**
discuss you with his friends within earshot?	**Red**

3. SOCIAL

Does he

point out boys you might like or girls he likes?	**Blue**
talk about places he'd like to take you?	**Pink**
ask when he can get you alone when you hardly know him?	**Red**

4. CONVERSATION

Does he

make crude comments?	**Red**

ask your opinion on things?	*Blue*
ask you about yourself?	*Pink*

5. FLIRTING
Does he

ignore your signals to back off and go more slowly?	*Red*
look into your eyes a lot and touch your arm?	*Pink*
ignore any flirting signals you send out?	*Blue*

6. OVERALL ATTITUDE
Does he

talk to you like he does his guy friends?	*Blue*
treat you with consideration and respect?	*Pink*
not seem to care what you think of his behavior?	*Red*

MAINLY BLUE: COOL CUSTOMER
Most likely explanation: this boy just wants to be friends. Bringing other people into your conversations shows he doesn't want your relationship to be exclusive. And if he's keeping his distance and not responding to your flirty advances, he's subtly making it clear that he's not interested. This gives you the chance to back off without possibly embarrassing yourself. Sorry. . .

But beware because: he could also be shy.

MAINLY RED: SCARY HORNDOG
Most likely explanation: this boy's up to no good. Grabbing your boobs, yelling to his friends about you, and making dirty remarks all show he has little respect for you and doesn't care whether you know it. Stick with him and you're in for heartache.

But beware because: he might just be too immature to know how to behave around girls.

MAINLY PINK: READY FOR ROMANCE

Most likely explanation: this boy's intentions are honorable. He sees a future with you and wants you to go places together. He cares about you and makes you feel special. He isn't all over you like a rash, but he gets close enough to show he's seriously attracted to you, and he doesn't want others to cut in while you're talking and spoil the vibe.

But beware because: he might be trying to manipulate you, particularly if he's older and more experienced.

The most important thing is to work out the finer points with each individual boy.

DATING

You like him and, as far as you can tell, he likes you. How do you get together? And what happens after that?

Asking Him Out

* **Don't** get your friend to ask him out for you. How on earth is the poor guy to know it's not a joke?
* **Do** try to get to know him a bit before you ask him out. If he responds well to you, make your move. Or keep bumping into him until he asks you!
* **Do** text him or ask him yourself. This is hard if you don't

know him at all, so your first task is to start talking to him.

* **Do** spend time with him in a group before you agree to pair off. That way there's less pressure to entertain each other. Plus you'll find out if you've got enough in common to see you through an hour or two alone together.

How to Have a Great Date

* **Don't** feel you have to be a one-stop entertainment shop and keep the conversation flowing all by yourself. A bit of silence is OK.

* **Do** ask him questions about his favorite subject—himself.

* **Don't** ask questions that can be answered yes or no. You need to get him talking.

* **Don't** let shyness kill the date stone dead. If you're self-conscious, concentrate on putting your boy at ease. This takes your mind off how well you think you're doing.

* **Don't** feel you have to go out in the evening. A daytime date feels more relaxed, so try a picnic in the park or a latte at a coffee shop.

* **Do** always tell someone—preferably a parent—where you are going.

* **Don't** knock back a few drinks to take the edge off your nerves. Booze can get you into potentially embarrassing and dangerous situations.

And Finally:
* **Don't** drop your friends every time a boy calls wanting to see you. Boys come and go, but a good friend is

always there with the Kleenex when he's ditched you for that flirty girl he met at the beach party.

Are You Ready to Date?

"Of course I am"! you scream, flinging this book across the room. But hold on to your hairdo. Yes, it might seem like everyone has a boyfriend, but feeling left out isn't a good enough reason to get one.

Everyone develops at different rates, and if you're really scared of boys, chances are you're a while away from being able to handle getting close to one. And that's OK. Hanging with friends who don't have boyfriends will stop you from feeling as though you've got two heads.

People who get into serious relationships young tend to go too far too soon because they don't have the emotional know-how to put the brakes on. Far better to wait until you know yourself better and have the confidence to say, "This is how I am. Take it or leave it, baby. There are plenty more fish in the sea!"

HAVING A BOYFRIEND

Pairing Up

So what happens when you get a boyfriend? Well, when you first start getting together with boys, relationships tend to be short. One started at lunchtime can be over by the next day. As you move further into your teens, generally you and one guy go from hanging with each other as part of a group to spending more time together alone. You share your hopes, fears, and dreams and enjoy feeling close and being there for each other.

You learn to negotiate when each of you sees your friends, how often you go out as a couple, and where you go. Then there's getting intimate: how far do you go and how fast? This hugely important and tricky subject will be covered in detail in part 3, "Sex and You." For now, here's how to manage the day-to-day relationship stuff.

Is It Love?

You've been out with your guy a few times and get along well, and you think you're really falling for him. Could this be love?

Is it obvious when you're in love? I get along great with this boy at school and feel all warm and tingly when we're together. Could I be in love with him? I asked my mom to explain what love is, but she couldn't. Help!

Caz, 14

Sorry to disappoint you, but I can't tell you exactly what love is either—even the experts have different definitions! Here are some pointers, though. Love, a crush, and lust (strong sexual desire) can all feel pretty similar, so it's only after quite a while that you can say, "Yes, this is love!" That's because real love lasts—it isn't over in three weeks.

Only by experiencing love can you get to know what it's like for you, but here's what other people have said it feels like. In the early stages, your heart thumps when the other person's near, you want to look at them and hug them and be with them all the time, and you seem to have so much in common that you talk nonstop. If the other person doesn't feel the same way, it's called a crush. So if you think you're falling for a boy big-time, the best advice is to enjoy what's happening between you, rather than trying to analyze it. Your feelings will become clear eventually.

Fights

When people first get together, they tend to be on their best behavior and try to please the other person. But the longer you're a couple, the more the differences between you will leak out. That's when the fights start, and some people think this is a sign the relationship should end. Not necessarily.

In all lasting relationships, we have to learn to negotiate with each other. Compromise is the key to successful relationships. So, for example, if he wants you to come watch a football game one Saturday, suggest that he come shopping with you the next week.

Getting Through Difficult Patches

* Negotiate: try and find solutions that involve compromise on both sides.

* Say what you mean rather than talking in code. For example, don't say, "Dave sure talks a lot, doesn't he?" when you really mean, "Can I see you without your friends more often?"

* Frame your complaints in terms of how you feel rather than blaming or insulting your partner. For example, "I feel left out when you talk to your friends and ignore me," rather than, "You're so selfish—you never think about me!"

Relationship-Wrecking Communication Styles

* *Withdrawal:* sulking or acting cold feels self-righteous because you're punishing the other person for hurting you. But it's manipulative and cruel: resist! If he's a sulker, leave him alone for a while to cool off. Pandering to sulkers only perpetuates the behavior.

* *Expecting the other person to read your mind.* However much he cares for you, he's not a mind reader, so *tell* him what you do or don't want.

* *Pretending to agree with what your partner's doing or saying when you really don't.* This might stop an argument for now, but the resentment will build, and you'll eventually blow.

Jealousy

This is a common problem, and it can be about anything: how much time one of you spends with friends, ogling a hottie in front of the other person, even lavishing so much attention on the dog that your beloved feels neglected. A touch of jealousy makes us feel loved, but constant suspicion and attempts to control the other person can be a huge problem.

If your partner's often jealous and you're not doing anything to provoke it, it's probably because he has difficulties with feeling secure that existed long before you came along—perhaps as a result of how his family treated him, so don't let him blame you for it. Keep your word if you agree to do something, but don't give in to all your boyfriend's demands, or the demands will become more and more unreasonable.

If you're the jealous one, remember that your boyfriend has a right to speak to others, just as you do, and that attempts to limit people's freedom generally backfire, causing them to

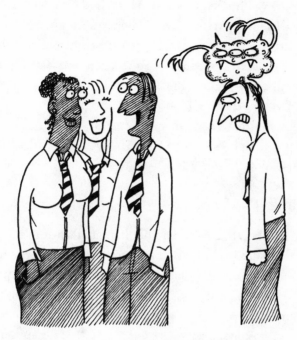

BEWARE! GREEN-EYED MONSTER!

leave. People who feel good about themselves are less likely to feel jealous, so follow the tips on pages 54–56 in "Boosting Your Self-Esteem."

Whether the green-eyed monster is you or your partner, counseling can help deep-rooted, destructive jealousy. See "Resources and Contacts" for ideas on finding a counselor locally.

To complicate matters further, there are people (and we can count many celebs among them) who, because of feelings of deep insecurity, have a desperate need to be the center of attention. For them, flirting and collecting admirers is a hobby, and many even enjoy the fact that it upsets their partner because that makes them feel even more wanted and important.

Compulsive flirters cause a lot of hurt, and their relationships rarely last, as most partners won't tolerate such poor treatment. If you recognize your boyfriend in this description, you can ask him to tone down his behavior, but it may be that his need for admiration overrides his feelings for you, and that's a shame. If you're the attention addict, recognize that there are other, less destructive ways to feel great. Again, check out "Boosting Your Self-Esteem" (pages 54–56) and consider talking to a counselor.

Two-Timing

If you're madly attracted to another person it's a sure sign that your relationship has run its course, so it makes sense to finish it completely before taking up with someone else. If a boy two-times his girlfriend with you and then dumps her for you, don't be too surprised when you get the same treatment down the line. Some two-timers get such a buzz from the deception that they'll do it over and over again.

Breaking Up

It's hard to do but, with most relationships, inevitable. You get bored, you fall for someone else, you discover you have less in common than you thought. If you want to get free of someone, do it quickly and cleanly and don't let them think they might still have a chance. Don't avoid them or act so rotten that they dump you. Treat them with the same respect you'd want in their place. Don't forget, you cared for them once.

Being dumped can be devastating (as if you didn't know). If this happens, don't search desperately for reasons, trying to work out what you did wrong. Accept that it's over and avoid your ex, as the longer you stay in contact, the longer it will take you to get over him. The loss can feel as bad as a bereavement, so cry as much as you need to and share your sad feelings with close friends and family. Keep busy and stay connected to the world. Soon you'll have filled the gap he left with other friends and interests, and eventually you'll be ready to date again.

Should I Get Back with Him?

This is one of the most commonly asked questions. The short answer is no (usually). It's tempting to slip back into a relationship that was as comfortable as a pair of old slippers, but nine times out of ten, the problems that cracked the relationship wide open the first time will still be there, and you'll break up again.

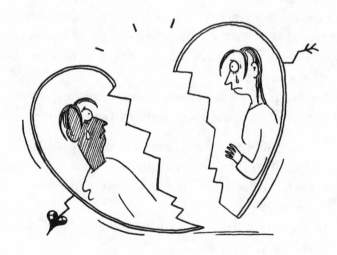

CHAPTER SIX
Sexuality

Even though you're not legally allowed to have sexual intercourse until you're a particular age, that doesn't mean you won't have sexual feelings before then. Sexual feelings can be really powerful and take you by surprise. When you're not used to them, it can seem like your body's running away with you and your hormones are turning you into a different person. Scary stuff!

The term *sex* is often used to mean sexual intercourse (penis in vagina), but it can also be used to refer to any sexual activity—for example, masturbation or contact with another person's genitals.

Loads of teenagers say that suddenly they can't stop thinking about sex and see it everywhere they look. This might not apply to you, or you may be somewhere in between. Guess what—it's all normal!

The first part of this chapter is made up of the questions I'm asked most often about sexual feelings. They are:

- What's this throbbing feeling between my legs?
- Could I go out with a celebrity?
- I'm turned on by pictures of women—what does it mean?
- Why do I fantasize about having sex?
- Will I ever want sex?
- What's cybersex?
- What do my sexy dreams mean?

After that, we move on to masturbation:

- What Is Masturbation?
- Masturbation Myths
- How Do Girls Masturbate?
- Why Do People Masturbate?
- Does Everyone Masturbate?

The rest of the chapter is about sexual orientation:

- Gay or Straight?
- Anti-Gay Feeling (Homophobia)

Common Questions About Sexuality

What's this throbbing feeling between my legs?

I sometimes get this throbbing feeling between my legs, which is weird, but nice. My seventeen-year-old girl cousin says it means I want to sleep with a boy. But I've never had a boyfriend and have only just started getting my period, so how can that be true?

If your cousin is sexually active, she's probably talking about what that feeling means to her. But in your case, what's happening is that you've reached the age when your body starts producing lots of the natural chemicals called hormones that make your breasts grow, your periods start, and your sexual organs mature. Hormones also affect your mind, and you can suddenly find yourself having lots of sexy thoughts. The throbbing you feel is probably because you've thought about or seen something sexy, like a guy you like, and have become a little sexually excited. If you were a boy, your penis would get stiff, but with girls, the tingly feelings are centered on the clitoris (a tiny, hooded pea-shaped organ at the top of your inner vaginal lips). It's all normal and isn't related to sexual experience. Your body is gearing up for when you're ready to get intimate either with yourself or another person.

Could I go out with a celebrity?

I know people say that they love celebrities, but this is different. I really do love this singer and I often imagine I'm kissing him. I'm sure we'd get along, so I want to meet him. I think about him night and day and cry over his posters. I hate school, but if I could go out with him all my problems would be solved.

It's perfectly natural to have strong feelings for a celeb. Most people fall for someone who's out of reach at some point, such as a teacher, an older boy, a celebrity, or even someone of their own sex. It's a safe way to experience the high of being in love, a kind of practice run for the real thing. And it feels like love—the difference is that the other person doesn't feel the same way. We're particularly likely to become infatuated when things aren't going well in our own lives, as it's such a pleasant distraction. If this describes you, enjoy your crush by all means, but try and remember that it's just that—a crush. Meanwhile, keep getting out there with your friends and in time you'll meet a boy with whom you can have an equal, loving relationship.

I'm turned on by pictures of women—what does it mean?

I get a kick out of looking at pictures of sexy women, and I've started to fantasize about being photographed for a porn magazine. I'm kind of scared of boys, though, and have never been asked out, so could I be a lesbian?

In your teens, it can suddenly seem like the world is full of sexy people, plus you start thinking of yourself as a potential sexual partner for someone. This is what a desire to be looked at in magazines is about —you want people to find you attractive. And they will, so try not to judge yourself harshly. Loads of teenagers find themselves attracted to people of the same sex, but whether you like boys or girls will become clear in time. For more on sexual orientation, see the section "Gay or Straight?" later in this chapter.

Why do I fantasize about having sex?

I've never even kissed a boy, but every night I lie in bed and imagine I'm doing sexy stuff with all sorts of people. I really enjoy these fantasies. Is this normal?

Yep! Many people, even the most unlikely ones, have sexual fantasies, and these can range from the perfectly ordinary to the downright bizarre. Fantasies can crop up when a person is masturbating or even when they're having sex with a partner. Sometimes men and women tell each other their fantasies as part of their sex life together. Fantasies are best when they remain just that, so take your time, and don't rush into anything sexwise. There's a very big difference between thinking sexy thoughts and making those thoughts a reality. And having sexy thoughts doesn't mean you're ready for sex.

Will I ever want sex?

I can't believe people enjoy sex. My friends are always talking about it, and I pretend to be interested, but the whole thing sounds absolutely disgusting. I don't think I'll ever want a boy to touch me. Am I a freak?

No—you're just at a different stage from your friends. Although lots of teenagers find the subject of sex endlessly fascinating, it's also perfectly normal not to want to join in. Plenty of people don't have much interest in sex until they fall in love, and then they find that sexual intimacy develops naturally out of their desire to express their feelings for the other person. And it may well be that you're the sort of person who prefers to keep their private life private, rather than putting your experiences on speakerphone. Instead of spending all your time with these people, perhaps it's time to find some friends who have interests other than sex.

What's cybersex?

When I was in a chat room recently I was asked to have cybersex by a boy my age who I really liked. What is cybersex, exactly? My cousin says she's done it but I don't dare ask her what it is.

On the Internet, chat rooms exist on every subject imaginable, and you can log on and chat with others by taking turns typing in replies. Most people who meet in chatrooms only communicate via computer and never meet face-to-face or even speak on the phone. Cybersex is where you and the person you're chatting with each masturbate yourselves (stroking the genital area until you have an orgasm) in front of your computers at the same time and type in how it feels. Or it can mean just talking about sexy stuff, without touching yourself. But if you're going to be sexual with someone, it's obviously better if it's a real person that you know well and can see and touch. The problem with meeting someone on the Internet is that you have no idea whether they're lying about their age, sex, and reason for chatting to you, and there are some very crazy people out there. You shouldn't meet up with people you contact this way for these reasons, nor should you give out personal details, such as your full name, address, or school. There's more on Internet safety in chapter 16.

What do my sexy dreams mean?

I keep having sexy dreams about all kinds of people I'm not attracted to in real life, such as my teachers, neighbors, and old film stars. What can I do to stop them? This can't be normal.

The bad news is that you have no control over what or who you dream about. The good news is that's OK, because it gives you permission to enjoy your sexy dreams without feeling guilty. There are lots of theories about dreams, but psychologists still don't know what our dreams are all about. Sigmund Freud thought they were partly concerned with wish fulfillment. Certainly with sexy dreams, which are very common, there's a part of us that is interested in sex and wants to experience sexual feelings, even though we may not be aware of it in our waking lives. Dreaming about intimate activities with someone doesn't necessarily mean you want to experience them in real life with that person.

MASTURBATION

What Is Masturbation?

Masturbation—rubbing your genital area until you have an orgasm—is a touchy subject (pardon the pun) that still upsets a lot of people. And yet we all touch ourselves between the legs from when we're tiny babies because it feels good. As we get older, we realize that some people disapprove, and we can then start to feel ashamed about handling our private areas. But for many young people, masturbation is a normal part of growing up and getting to know their own body.

Masturbation Myths

There are tons of these, but here are the most common:

Masturbation . . .

- *gives you pimples;*
- *makes you crazy;*
- *makes you blind;*
- *stunts your growth;*
- *reduces your chances of becoming a parent;*
- *makes a girl's clitoris grow or leads to other genital deformities;*
- *means you won't enjoy sex with another person.*

All of these are utterly untrue.

Boys tend to masturbate more than girls and start earlier, and there are several reasons for this. Boys generally have more contact with their genitals than do girls. For example, they handle their penises every day when they pee, and they soon discover how nice it feels to touch them in certain ways. And society is much stricter with girls about every aspect of their sexuality, making them more likely to feel bad about sexy feelings. But we're all different.

> *I'm worried there's something wrong with me because I masturbate whenever I get a sexy thought, which is pretty often. My best friend was shocked when I told her this and says she's never touched herself. Will I always be like this?*
>
> Angie, 14

Some girls never masturbate, others do it occasionally, and yet others do it every day—it's up to the individual. It's a good way of finding out what feels best, information that you can share with a partner when the time comes. It's quite common to masturbate a lot when you first discover how to do it.

Everyone's sex drive is different, but plenty of women still masturbate regularly in adulthood, even when they have a long-term partner. If you're generally happy with your life and masturbate a lot, then you probably just have a high sex drive. But occasionally, it can be that you spend a lot of time touching yourself as a distraction from difficult areas of your life, and if that's the case, you need to take some time to look for solutions.

How Do Girls Masturbate?

Most boys tend to masturbate in the same way—by rubbing their hand up and down their penis until they ejaculate (come). For girls it's rather different. Some girls can orgasm from breast stimulation alone, while others can do it just by squeezing their thighs together. But most need to stimulate their clitoris to have an orgasm, and do this with their fingers, with a jet of water from a hand-held showerhead, with a vibrator (a battery-operated device, often shaped a bit like a penis), or by rubbing against something soft like a pillow. Often one side of the clitoris is more sensitive than the other.

Some prefer to have something inside their vagina too, like their fingers, but if you like to do this, make sure you don't use anything with sharp edges or that could break inside you, such as a glass object.

Why Do People Masturbate?

Some of the reasons people masturbate are:

- because they're feeling turned on;
- to release tension;
- to help them sleep;
- to learn what an orgasm feels like;
- to get to know their body;
- as part of lovemaking with a partner.

Does Everyone Masturbate?

No. You might not feel the need to do it. For some of us, the messages we've absorbed from those around us means we just don't feel comfortable with masturbation, and that's OK too. It doesn't mean you won't be able to enjoy sex when the right person comes along. Some people never masturbate, while others do throughout their life, and still others only do so occasionally.

GAY OR STRAIGHT?

I was showering with my schoolmates after swimming one day when I suddenly found I couldn't stop staring at their bodies. That night I found myself picturing what I'd seen and getting turned on. I've got a boyfriend, so I don't think I'm a lesbian, but could I be bisexual?

Meera, 15

This is a natural reaction. When we first start to encounter sexual feelings, we look for people to attach them to. Because we spend much more time with people of our own sex, we feel closer to them, and it's easy for these feelings to turn sexual.

Gay (also called homosexual) people are attracted to their own sex, straight (heterosexual) ones like the opposite sex, and bisexuals are attracted both to their own and the opposite sex. This is called your sexual orientation. No conclusive study exists, but it's estimated that between five and ten in every hundred people are gay. Some boys and girls lust after people of their own sex and end up being gay, but others are attracted to people of the opposite sex when they're young and still end up gay. And while some people are sure they're gay from very early on, others don't realize it until they're in their late teens or twenties, or sometimes even older.

As a teenager, it's common to be attracted to or even experiment with your own sex and still end up straight, so if this happens to you, try not to slap a label on yourself. You can take as long as you like to find out what you feel inside—no one's holding a stopwatch.

If you're worried about any feelings you have in this area, find someone you trust to talk them over with. If that's not possible, or you want to discuss this with a trained counselor who understands exactly what you're going through and won't judge you, call the National Gay and Lesbian Youth Hotline at 1-800-347-TEEN.

Anti-Gay Feeling (Homophobia)

Despite plenty of research, we still don't know what makes a person gay, straight, or bisexual. But plenty of "straight" people are frightened and shocked at the thought of homosexuality, and some even believe it's an illness. Pedophiles (adults who sexually abuse children) have been in the news a lot recently, and it's sometimes wrongly thought that most pedophiles are gay men. Actually, the vast majority of men who abuse children are heterosexuals targeting young girls.

Lesbians and gay men face discrimination in their lives, from being denied privileges that straight people get automatically to being called hurtful names or beaten up—all because of who they're attracted to.

Luckily, society as a whole is becoming more tolerant of those who are different. As more people stand up and say they're gay—including those in the public eye and the media— and education and other institutions become more inclusive, it's getting easier for the rest of us to accept such feelings if we have them, and for our family and friends to accept them too.

CHAPTER SEVEN
Attitudes Toward Sex

Your values are a big part of who you are. Take lying, for example. Perhaps you believe it's OK to tell a white lie to save someone's feelings. Or that there's nothing wrong in telling whoppers to get you off the hook. Or maybe you think that lying for any reason is out of order. We all have to work out where we stand on life's big stuff, and in the world of sex and relationships, what you do or don't believe has major consequences.

It takes a lifetime to work out your codes and values, but your teenage years are when you really start to notice and question others' beliefs. To make matters even more confusing, there are plenty of contradictory messages. For example, despite daily cooking shows featuring mouth-watering, fattening dishes and the barrage of ads for fast-food outlets, we're supposed to ignore them and choose salads because they're better for us. We're told to hold out for our one true love, yet some celebs change their partners almost as often as their clothes. Girls believe they should look and act sexy to catch a boy's eye, but if they have sex, they're often called sluts. What's a girl to think?

To help you, this chapter looks at the main influences on our values and attitudes about sex:

- Parents
- Religion and Culture
- The Media
- Friends

- School
- Sex and the Law: Legal Age of Consent; Prosecution for Underage Sex; Gay and Lesbian Sex; Porn; Sex for Money (Prostitution)
- Your Values

PARENTS

Once you become aware of your own sexual feelings, it might suddenly dawn on you that your parents must have done the deed to produce you—yuck! But what your parents think has a huge influence on how you feel about sex and relationships. No matter what they say about the male-female stuff (if they say anything at all!), it's how they behave, which you'll have been absorbing since you were knee-high to a grasshopper, that affects you the most.

A good example is teenage motherhood. If your mom had you as a young teenager, your chances of repeating this in your own life are high, despite no doubt getting grim warnings of how hard it is and how much your mom regrets starting a family so young. This is partly because, from your earliest years, you soaked up like a sponge the idea: *This is how our family does motherhood.*

If your dad treats your mom with courtesy and respect, you're likely to expect this in your own relationships. Or if you live with one parent who can't sort out his or her relationships, you may find it harder to trust a partner than someone who's been brought up by two parents who are committed to each other.

Parents who show affection to you and each other and make it clear that they have a fulfilling sex life (sorry!) give you the

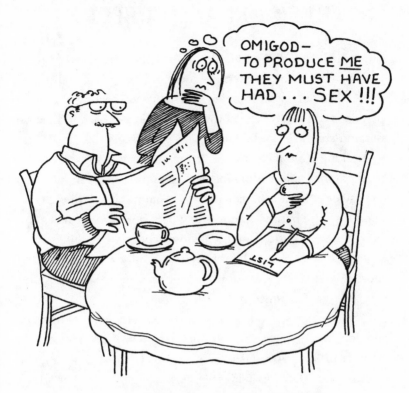

PARENTS — THE TRUTH

unspoken message that sex is a good thing and that you're a lovable person who can expect the same kind of relationship for yourself. Parents sleeping in separate beds or slapping your hand away when you're little if it creeps near your genitals send the message: *Our family doesn't do sex.*

Survey after survey shows that teenagers say they'd love to be able to talk frankly to their parents about sex and relationships. For tips on how to approach the old folks about this tricky subject, turn to chapter 13.

RELIGION AND CULTURE

There are lots of different faiths and beliefs in the United States, each of which has its own ideas about sex and sexuality and what behavior is acceptable. And while respecting the other person is central to most of them, the beliefs of each individual religion about sex and relationships vary hugely.

Seeking guidance from your religious leaders, talking to your parents, and reading the texts of your religion should help to answer your questions within your faith. This is all well and good if you're happy to adhere to what your faith preaches and find it fits in with your own moral codes. Difficulties arise when the culture or religion of your family clashes with the more liberal Western attitudes and behavior you see all around you, and you're pulled in two directions.

The most common examples are where your culture or religion frowns upon sex before marriage or marrying outside your faith, and you wish to do one or both of those things. Sharing your feelings with friends, teachers, and other adults you trust may help, but there are no easy answers. In the "Resources and Contacts" section you might find a service that can help you work through the issues. Alternatively, there are support groups for almost everything, many of which can be found on the Internet. If you do seek help on the Internet, as always, never give out personal details such as your name, address, phone number, or school.

Ultimately, when you're eighteen and an adult, you can make your own choices independent of your family. This will be hard if they're opposed to your decisions, so it will help if you can create a network of likeminded people to support you.

THE MEDIA

It's already been mentioned in the chapter on body image how the media hold up visions of women rendered "perfect" by cosmetic surgery, clever styling, crash diets, and, when all else fails, airbrushing out their remaining blemishes in photos, and how bad ordinary girls feel when they can't get anywhere near meeting these impossible standards.

On top of this, soap operas, films, billboards, music videos, magazines, and ads make it seem like this never-ending parade of beautiful people spend their lives half-naked and pairing off with other hotties.

Unless you live on a desert island, it's impossible not to be affected by this constant bombardment of sexy images. You might easily find yourself getting a little turned on umpteen times a day by the time you've seen X's six-pack flexing across a magazine cover; Y's glossy, bikini-clad body on a billboard advertising soap; P and Q cavorting on a sofa in *Desperate Housewives*; and Z's erotic dance to his latest song on MTV. It's easy to end up thinking, "Everybody's doing it, so why shouldn't I be too?"

But they're not. It's an illusion based on the fact that, as a strong drive, sex will always have the power to make people sit up and take notice. Lots of us get a quick buzz from admiring the good-looking people the media shove in our faces, but then go back, quite happily, to our ordinary, everyday lives. The older you get, the less you're affected by the standards of perfection perpetuated by the media and the more content you'll be with who you are. Honestly!

FRIENDS

Friends, eh? Who'd we be without 'em? When you're growing up and learning to be independent of your family, your friends become a vital source of support and guidance. It's really important to feel liked and accepted by groups we look up to, and sometimes we find ourselves doing things we'd prefer not to so we'll fit in. Being different from the crowd in any way can lead to teasing and bullying, so it's no wonder it's hard to go with the flow of your own feelings if they're not the same as your friends'.

Where sex is concerned, lots of teenagers cave in and do it not because they really want to, but because of outside pressure. Boys are more likely to lose their virginity because of peer pressure from their friends. Girls are more likely to succumb to heavy-handed tactics from a boyfriend. (See chapter 13 on how to deal with pressure from boyfriends.)

And getting a boyfriend just because your friends have one isn't a good basis for a relationship. You'll be more concerned with comparing notes with your friends than forging a loving, trusting relationship, which isn't fair to the guy. Being single gives you more of a chance to get to know yourself and work on your goals and talents, so make the most of it.

SCHOOL

Many people believe that sex education makes teenagers more likely to rush out and lose their virginity at an early age, but research shows that the opposite is true. Young people for whom sex ed is their main source of info on sex tend to lose their virginity later than those who say friends and the media are their primary source.

Unfortunately, not all schools are equally good when it comes to sex ed. Lots of you report being disappointed by it, saying that it's too biological and there's not enough emphasis on emotions and feelings. According to a recent teen magazine survey, 60 percent of readers say sex education in their school is "not good." Your parents have the right to take you out of any portion of sex ed that they aren't comfortable with, although most don't do this.

Of course, you also get messages about sex and relationships at school informally from other pupils, from the values of the school, and from how your teachers deal with the subject.

SEX AND THE LAW

Legal Age of Consent

The laws about underage sex exist to protect young people until they're mature enough to make their own decisions about who they have sex with. In the United States, the age at which you can legally engage in heterosexual sex is different from state to state. With a few exceptions, the legal age of consent is between sixteen and eighteen.

Prosecution for Underage Sex

Technically it's a criminal offense for two people to have any kind of sexual contact under the age of consent. In reality, as long as both parties agreed to sex, there's not much difference in their ages, and there's no evidence that one partner exploited the other, it's highly unlikely that teens will be prosecuted. This law is meant to protect young people from harm and exploitation by adults.

Gay and Lesbian Sex

In the United States, each state has its own laws about homosexual acts. For a state-by-state listing, go to http://www.ageofconsent.com.

Porn

Pornography consists of images, books, or films whose sole purpose is to make people sexually aroused. The laws surrounding pornography are muddy in that sexually explicit images are legal, but if something is considered obscene, which means likely to "deprave" and "corrupt," it's illegal. This has to be decided by a court, but some types of porn, such as child pornography, are illegal in any form.

Given that sexually explicit images are in demand, the porn industry makes some people very rich, and now that images can be distributed via the Internet, it's growing faster than ever.

Pornography provokes strong feelings both for and against it. Some feel it should all be banned, while at the opposite end of the spectrum, others believe that any form of censorship is wrong. As most porn is produced for heterosexual men, one argument is that it degrades the women who appear in the pictures and films, while others argue that it's their choice to do so.

Porn isn't meant to be realistic—the whole point is to turn people on. Sex therapists (professionals who help people overcome problems with their sex lives) may suggest to their clients that they read sexy stories, look at porn mags, or watch a porn video as part of their "homework." Ultimately, it's up to you to decide what you think about porn. If your boyfriend looks at porn and you're worried about this, see page 111.

Sex for Money (Prostitution)

Most prostitutes are women who have sex with men for money, although there are gay male prostitutes who sell sex to men and a tiny number of men who sell sex to women. Except in Nevada, prostitution is illegal throughout the United States.

Paying for sex obviously doesn't involve a close, caring, and equal relationship, and plenty of people believe it's morally wrong. However, our society has muddled ideas about the link between sex and money. For example, often we see older, rich men marrying younger, attractive women, and the women see this as a fair trade-off. And unfortunately sometimes a boy might think he's entitled to a kiss, a grope, or even full sex if he paid to take you on a date. It goes without saying that he most certainly is NOT. You should never feel obliged to be intimate with anyone, for whatever reason.

YOUR VALUES

This chapter will have given you some idea of how your family, religion and culture, the media, your friends, school, and the law might influence your thinking about sex and relationships. The key to learning how to make your own decisions in these and other areas is to find out as much as you can from reliable sources, think things through, and discuss any questions with a trusted adult. Some decisions you'll be happy with, others less so. Some you might even regret, but each one will teach you more about what you consider acceptable and unacceptable.

CHAPTER EIGHT
Emotions Q & A

Stand by for your most-asked questions about your emotional life. They are:

- Why is there a legal age to have sex?
- My best friend has had sex—should I?
- How do you date?
- How can I persuade my parents to let me see him?
- How can we get around our families' religious differences?
- Does she want me as a friend or a lover?
- How can I catch this older guy?
- Are all boys sex-crazed?
- Why does my boyfriend look at porn?
- Which boys are genuine?

Why is there a legal age to have sex?
I don't understand why it's against the law to have sex under the legal age limit. I'm fourteen, and two of the girls in my class have slept with their boyfriends, who are the same age. Could they all go to prison?

It *is* against the law to have sexual intercourse under the age of sixteen in most U.S. states, but, in reality, if two young teenagers are around the same age and both want to have sex, it's extremely unlikely that anyone will be prosecuted. When you're young, your dating experiences tend to be pretty short and you might have lots of quick relationships. By the age of fifteen or sixteen, though, a person's increasing emotional maturity means they have a growing sense of commitment and responsibility. This means they're more able to stick with a relationship and get to know and trust their partner, both essential elements of a successful sexual relationship. Sex stirs up powerful emotions, and to deal with them you need to know yourself well. Of course, you're not necessarily mature when you reach your sixteenth or eighteenth birthday, but these are considered the minimum ages a person will be aware of what a sexual relationship means. But this doesn't mean you have to be ready for sex at a specific age. And why hurry? So try not to let the girls at school influence you—find out the facts and decide for yourself.

My best friend has had sex—should I?

My best friend and I go out with boys who are also best friends, and my friend recently lost her virginity to her boyfriend. Now all three say it's time I slept with my boyfriend. I'm not sure, but I'm worried that my friend is in a more grown-up relationship than I am and I don't want to feel left out.

I'd say, "You might be a bunch of sheep, but I make my own decisions and I'm not ready for sex!" It may actually be that your friend regrets what she did and wants you to have sex to make her feel better about herself. You may see her as more grown up, but the fact that you're trying to resist pressure and thinking for yourself shows that you're the more mature one. Perhaps you could point out that if she does wish she hadn't gone all the way, she doesn't *have* to have sex again. And if you see life as a competition where you must be at the same stage or ahead of your friends, you'll find yourself doing all kinds of things you don't want to, for appearances' sake. Stand firm and you'll find the people who matter will respect you for making up your own mind.

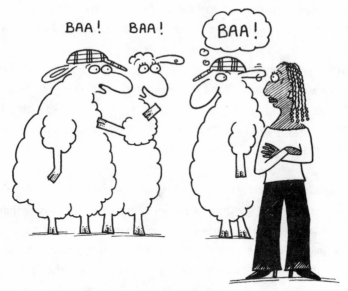

How do you date?

I have two sisters and I go to an all-girls' school, so I haven't a clue how to talk to boys, but I'd love to go on dates now that I'm sixteen. I don't go out very often, but where do boys hang out?

Forget about dating for now. Before dating comes friendship, so make your priority finding some male friends. Once you're comfortable spending time with guys, then you can start thinking about boyfriends. Maybe one of the guys you become friendly with might end up as something more. If you don't go out much, you're probably short on female friends too, so perhaps your problem is more about loneliness in general than lack of a boyfriend. To kick-start your social life, visit your local library and ask for a list of what's happening in your area for teenagers. Whatever your interests—sports, music, books—there'll be a club for it, so join up. Get people talking about themselves, become a good listener, and treat them with respect. Making friends is daunting at first, but if you practice, you'll be fine.

How can I persuade my parents to let me see him?

My mom found my boyfriend's condoms at our house, and she's banned me from seeing him now that she knows we have sex. Because my boyfriend is seventeen and I'm only fifteen, my parents have threatened to have him prosecuted for sleeping with me, unless I do as they say. My boyfriend's evening job means he's free in the daytime, so I cut school to see him. I don't want to deceive my parents, but I just don't know what else to do.

The way to get what you want from your parents is to show them you can act responsibly. Cutting school brings more problems than it solves because your teachers will tell your parents and then they'll trust you even less—with good reason. And if your parents think it's irresponsible for a boy of seventeen to sleep with a fifteen-year-old girl, imagine how furious they'll be with him when they find out he encourages you to miss school too. As you're underage, it's possible that your boyfriend could be prosecuted for sleeping with you, so it would be better to stop the sex altogether, have contact with your boyfriend just by phone for now, and get back to school. Your parents may be angry, but the more they see you following their rules, the sooner they'll trust you enough to let you out. Sometimes one parent is easier to talk to, and if you're able to win the support of that parent, he or she will argue your case to the other one. Perhaps they'd be willing to meet your boyfriend. If they get to know him, they may let you see him, even if it's only at your house at first.

How can we get around our families' religious differences?

I'm a Muslim girl, and I've got a fantastic boyfriend who's Hindu. We've been talking about getting married as soon as we can. His parents are cool about me not being Hindu, but although mine let us meet up at school, they insist that when I marry, it must be to another Muslim. How can I get them to understand my point of view? My boyfriend and I are both fifteen.

It's very hard when your family abides by cultural values that feel uncomfortable to you as a young person growing up in the United States. You want to please your family but also want to be happy with your choice of partner. Every state has its own law, but in most states you can get married from the age of sixteen, with your parents' consent. When you're eighteen, you can marry whoever you like (unless you live in Nebraska or Mississippi, where you're required to be older), although it might still be hard to go against your family's wishes. Having said that, fifteen is awfully young to be thinking about marriage. You need to be careful not to rush into things just to spite your parents. How about trying to enjoy the time you spend with your boyfriend instead of worrying about the future? Meanwhile, find someone in your family or religious community to confide in about this. It may be that your parents will come to terms with the idea in time, especially if they get to know and like your boyfriend. You may also find that, as you get older, your parents are more willing to listen to your point of view.

Does she want me as a friend or a lover?

This girl recently moved in on my street and we've been seeing a lot of each other. But the other day she put a note through my door, saying she's a lesbian, and since then I've been avoiding her because I'm scared that she plans to make a move on me. I miss her as a friend, though—what should I do?

Your worry is a common one: that gay people have sexual feelings toward everyone who's the same sex as them. Well, it's not true. Just like you don't like every boy you meet, gay people are attracted to certain individuals and not to others. Up to ten in every hundred people are gay. Even so, fear and prejudice mean that gay people are frequently treated in ways that are hurtful, and it was probably quite hard for your friend to tell you she's a lesbian. So don't add to any unkindness she may already have been subjected to by ignoring her. That will upset both of you. Why not ask her a bit about how she found out she was attracted to girls, and make it clear you like boys? If she does turn out to like you then, yes, it would make friendship difficult. But if you just avoid her, you may lose a good friend for nothing.

How can I catch this older guy?

This gorgeous twenty-year-old guy works at the gas station near my house and I can't stop thinking about him. I'd do anything to be near him, and even if he won't go out with me, I'd be happy just to be his friend. He's nice to me but changes the subject when I ask for his number. What am I doing wrong? I'm fifteen—might he think I'm too young?

OK, say you're friends with him and one day, you bump into him with a girl. "Hi," he says, "meet my new girlfriend." Would you be cool about that? Thought not. Fact is, it's very common to have crushes on people we can't have. Older guys are particularly attractive, as they seem so interesting and smart compared to boys your age. Crushes are a practice run for falling in love for real. You get the highs and lows, but from a safe distance. It seems cruel, but this guy is behaving responsibly by not encouraging you. Drool over him from afar by all means, but be aware it won't come to anything, including friendship. Meanwhile, get out and about with boys nearer your own age.

EMOTIONS Q & A

Are all boys sex-crazed?

I really want a boyfriend, but the boys in my area only go out with girls for the sex, and if you don't give it to them, they'll find someone else who will. My friends and I want to know if all boys are the same. It's so depressing.

There's an awful lot of pressure on boys to prove to their friends how "manly" they are, and unfortunately an accepted way of doing this is by racking up sexual partners. Plus, girls mature emotionally earlier than boys, and so are ready for committed relationships at a younger age. But this does change as boys get into their late teens and twenties, so don't despair. Meanwhile, there are boys your age who aren't just after sex, and they're easy to spot because they treat you with respect from the start and don't grope you against your will.

Why does my boyfriend look at porn?

My boyfriend's closet was open the other day and I noticed a pile of porn mags in the bottom. What on earth does he want these for? I'm horrified, but I'm not sure what to say to him.

Pornography is sexy material, such as pictures and videos, that's intended to sexually arouse people. Naked women feature heavily in pornography. It's used mainly by men because they tend to be excited by visual images, while women are more likely to prefer sexy fantasies. While some men share porn with their partners, most use it to turn themselves on and masturbate to, which is what your boyfriend is probably doing. Such magazines aren't for sale to people under eighteen, so their forbidden nature makes them even more attractive to young men. Your boyfriend isn't alone. The occasional look at a girlie mag won't do any harm. In fact, some sex therapists give "soft" porn to people with sexual problems to help them learn how to get turned on. The problem comes if a person becomes so addicted to porn that he (or she) prefers it to real-life relationships, which doesn't seem to apply to your boyfriend. However, you have every right to disagree with your boyfriend about this, so it sounds like you need to tell him how it makes you feel. Hopefully he'll take your feelings into consideration, but ultimately you can't stop him from using porn. If he refuses to give it up, you'll have to decide whether you're still prepared to see him.

Which boys are genuine?

Boys have asked me out before, but when I said yes, it turned out they were only joking. Now I don't dare agree to a date, but some of these boys might be serious. How can I tell who to trust?

You can't tell up front if you can trust a person. The only way to find out if a boy is reliable is to get to know him and see how he behaves toward you. And that means you have to let go of some of your suspiciousness and trust him a little. You don't have to start off with real dates—see how it goes as friends first. Trustworthiness is the sum total of lots of kinds of behavior. Important elements of trust are being on time for dates, keeping promises, telling the truth, and keeping the intimate details of your relationship secret. A reliable boyfriend will do all these things, which show he's treating you with respect and consideration. There are plenty of decent boys out there, so why not use your instincts to pick a boy and give him a chance!

PART THREE

Sex and You

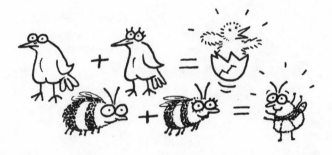

CHAPTER NINE

Are You Ready for Sex?

Deciding that you want to have sexual intercourse, with all the risks and responsibilities that it brings, is a major step in your life. There's no rush to have sex—you can still enjoy life, love, and boys—but it's important to be informed. And in this section, hopefully you'll find the answers to all your questions on sex itself, boys and sex, contraception, and sexual health. Toward the end of the book, you'll find chapters on unwanted sexual attention and pregnancy. If you need further information, you'll find a list of organizations than can help at the back of the book.

Taking things a step at a time, chapter 9 asks the vital question: are you ready for sexual intercourse?

So how *do* you know when you're ready? Only you can decide that, but in this chapter are some ideas about:

- Virginity
- Waiting to Have Sex
- Right Time, Right Person
- Questions to Ask Yourself
- Bad Reasons for Having Sex
- Regrets

VIRGINITY

Although it can seem like everyone you know is having sex, they're really not. Research shows that the average age for first-time sex is 16.9 years for boys and 17.4 years for girls, so there are a lot of teenagers out there who are still virgins.

The only way to lose your virginity is by having penetrative sex—this is when the boy puts his penis in the girl's vagina. Tampons, exploring fingers, and hymens broken through exercise don't count—you're still a virgin until that's happened. Technically it's generally agreed that, sexist as it is, your first experience of intercourse is over when the boy has ejaculated (come). But if a boy's penis is only inside you for a little while, or it doesn't go all the way in, or he doesn't come, it's up to you to decide whether you'e still a virgin or not.

Some people think of virginity as a barrier between childhood and adulthood to be crashed through at the first opportunity. But having sex doesn't make you a mature adult. That comes with time, experience, knowing and understanding yourself, and being able to stop and think of the consequences before rushing into situations, however much you might want to go ahead. But although the law about having to be sixteen to eighteen for sex, depending on the state, may seem old-fashioned, it's there for good reasons. Studies show that people under sixteen are less likely to use contraception and more likely to regret having sex. So, just because you *want* to have sex doesn't necessarily mean you're ready to.

Losing your virginity is a very special experience. You'll remember your first time forever, so it makes sense for it to be with someone you care for deeply and who cares for you. Even if you're no longer with the person, it's better to be able to look back with a warm glow rather than shuddering and trying to push the event to the back of your mind. Once you've gone all the way with someone, you can't go back. And a really awful first time can put you off sex for years.

WAITING TO HAVE SEX

One study of sixteen- to twenty-four-year-olds who've had sex found that two in ten of the boys and four in ten of the girls wished they'd waited longer before losing their virginity. And the younger you are when you have sex, the more likely you are to regret it.

We'd done other stuff together, and sex just seemed like the next step. Although I liked Jason, I didn't really love him, but I wanted to find out what sex was like. I've been with my fantastic boyfriend Dez for nearly a year now, and I really wish I'd waited so I could have shared that first experience with him.

Ashley, 17

Leroy had slept with other girls, and I felt silly saying no, as he was so experienced. I was a virgin and said I wanted to wait, but he was pushy so I went ahead in the end. He dumped me a week later. I felt like such an idiot.

Petra, 16

I'd only been with Simon two weeks, but we ended up getting drunk at my best friend's party and it just happened. We'd never talked about contraception and didn't have any condoms. I was so scared I was pregnant that I went on and on about it until my period came. By then, Simon was so sick of me ranting that the relationship just fell apart.

Joely, 16

Most teenagers who regret having sex feel they weren't emotionally ready. Often they were doing it because their partner or friends said they should.

You might have strong religious, cultural, or personal reasons not to have sex yet or to wait until you're married. You have every right to hold such views, so don't let anyone convince you otherwise. If you go against these views and have sex anyway, you're going to feel you've let yourself and probably your family down. Is it really worth it?

The risks that come with sex—muddled emotions, pregnancy, and sexually transmitted diseases—are very serious and are there from the very first time you have sex. You'll also need an armory of defenses at the ready to back up your decision if you decide to go against your partner's wishes and say no. Turn to chapter 13 for tips on how to deal with this assertively.

Even if you really are the last virgin your age in your hometown, then good for you for refusing to run with the pack. If anyone tries to make you feel bad about it, it's your call to tell them to mind their own business and then feel super smug for making your own decisions.

RIGHT TIME, RIGHT PERSON

Sex can generate incredibly strong emotions, and it's true that having sex with someone you love deeply and who feels the same way about you is probably one of the most rewarding, fulfilling experiences life has to offer. But, unfortunately, sex with the wrong person can be one of the most humiliating and upsetting things that will ever happen to you, so it's important to get it right if you can. And the final decision *is* up to you, whatever anyone says.

Sixteen to eighteen (depending on where you live) is the age at which you can legally have sex, but there isn't a magic age when you're ready for sex—we all mature at different rates. Reaching either of these ages doesn't automatically mean you should have sex just because you can. The emotional maturity needed to cope with the responsibilities and commitments of a sexual relationship doesn't land on your doormat along with your birthday cards. It's OK to wait.

Getting intimate with someone you really like doesn't have to be about full-on sex anyway. You can have a great time kissing, touching, and cuddling!

QUESTIONS TO ASK YOURSELF

If you're thinking of having sex, ask yourself the following questions:

- *Am I legal?* Technically, sexual intercourse under the age of sixteen or eighteen (depending upon where you live) isn't legal. And the younger you have sex, the more risk there is of regretting it. Is it worth it?
- *Can I say the words* condom, penis, vagina, *and* sex *without cracking up or turning beet red?* If you don't feel comfortable discussing the basics of sex, you're definitely not ready to do it. The best experiences come after you and your partner have, over time, told each

other your hopes and fears about sex and planned it properly, including contraception and protection against diseases.

- *Am I confident enough to buy condoms or ask for them at a clinic, and talk to a doctor or nurse about contraception?* You have a responsibility to protect yourself and your partner from pregnancy and sexually transmitted diseases.

- *Do I understand the basics of how pregnancy happens, how contraception works, and how sexually transmitted diseases are passed on?* This is absolutely vital pre-sex knowledge.

- *Do I know my partner well and trust that he'd stop if I said no, even at the last minute?* You need to be able to trust him completely and to have discussed this possibility ahead of time. Remember, it's your right to refuse to go further at any point.

- *Do I feel strongly about him and care for him, and does he feel the same about me?* You both need to make sure that your partner is OK before, during, and after sex, and if one of you isn't interested in the other as a person, that won't happen. Also, if things go wrong and there is a pregnancy or an STD, you need to be able to decide what to do together and rely on each other for support.

- *Is my partner putting pressure on me to have sex?* If you're doing this to please the other person, not because you want to, you're likely to regret it.

- *Has my partner ever said or implied that he'd break up with me if I don't sleep with him?* If so, chances are he's either so focused on the sex that he's lost sight of you as a person, or he's into scoring sex points and doesn't much care who it's with. Whatever the reason, a boy who respects his girlfriend and wants the relationship to continue wouldn't dare threaten her.

- *Have I tried other sexual things with my boyfriend, and do I feel turned on?* If your body doesn't respond to your partner, you're not ready to go on to full sex.
- *Am I happy for him to see me naked?* The days of Victorian ladies doing it through a hole in their nighties are long gone. If you're too shy to take off at least some of your clothes, forget it for now.
- *Do I know about the various different types of sex—for example, oral and full penetrative intercourse—and the risks of each?* See chapters 11 and 18 for info on these.
- *Does sex at this time fit in with my personal, religious, or cultural values?* Again, you're likely to regret it if not.
- *Do I know how my parents feel about me having sex?* You may not want to talk to them about it right away, but you may need their support in the future, so it's best to have an idea how they'd react. If they think you're too young, give their views some serious thought rather than dismissing them outright.
- *Am I ready to say good-bye to the virgin part of me?* Having sex will change the way you see yourself, but you won't know exactly how until afterward.
- *Do I have any doubts at all about going ahead?* If so, stop right there and wait until you're certain.

Yes, it's an awesome checklist, but the more of these you can answer truthfully and satisfactorily, the more likely it is that you're ready to go ahead.

Bad Reasons for Having Sex

We've looked at some of the questions you might want to consider before having sex. What about negative reasons for jumping into bed?

Are You Considering Sex . . .

* To see what it's like?
* To "get rid" of your virginity?
* To see if you can do it?

You'll have plenty of sex in your life if that's what you want, so what's the hurry? And unless you've been born without a vagina or penis, everyone can have sex, so relax!

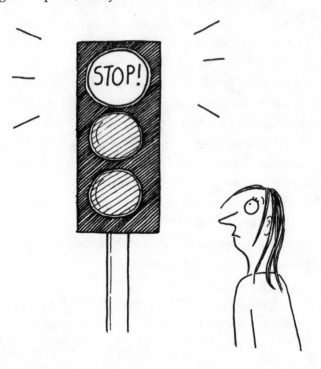

Or . . .

* Because the other person expects it?
* To prove you love someone?

Sleeping with someone against your better judgment only proves that the other person is a master of emotional blackmail. Always remember that your feelings are as valid as anyone else's.

Or . . .

* To be just like your friends?

If they all jumped off the Brooklyn Bridge with their underwear on their heads, would you? Lots of your friends will be exaggerating anyway. Go at your own pace and ignore what everyone else claims they're doing.

Or . . .

* Because you're drunk or on drugs?

Being so out of it that you've got no control over what you're doing is a recipe for being used and abused, or doing something you'll later wish you hadn't.

Regrets

But, as a famous musician (John Lennon, if you must know) once said, life is what happens to you while you're busy making other plans. You weighed the pros and cons and did your utmost to be sensible, but one thing led to another and—you did it. And now you wish you hadn't.

As much as I've been going on about safeguarding yourself against regretting having sex, beating yourself up from now until you draw your last breath won't change anything, so lay off. We all do things we wish we hadn't, and the best advice is to have a good cry with your best friend, chalk it up to experience, forgive yourself, and move on.

But if you're really distressed, see "Resources and Contacts" for who to turn to for help.

CHAPTER TEN

Contraception

Part of being ready to take your relationship further and have penetrative sex is being mature enough to use contraception to protect against unwanted pregnancy. Sexual contact can also result in catching or passing on diseases, including HIV, the virus that causes AIDS, so it's vital to know how to guard yourself and your partner against sexually transmitted diseases (STDs) too.

STDs are covered in chapter 11. This chapter covers:

- Contraception—What's It All About?: Where to Go for Contraception; Myths About Preventing Pregnancy; Natural Method
- Methods of Contraception: Condoms; Combination Pill; Progestin-Only Pill (POP or Mini-Pill); Contraceptive Injections; Diaphragms and Caps; Intrauterine Devices; The Contraceptive Patch
- Emergency Contraception: What Is Emergency Contraception?; Method One: Emergency Contraceptive Pills; Method Two: IUD

CONTRACEPTION: WHAT'S IT ALL ABOUT?

Contraception means "against conception": stopping sexual intercourse from leading to pregnancy using natural or man-made methods. The first U.S. birth control clinic appeared in 1916, but was raided by a vice squad ten days later. Luckily, society has changed a lot since then. Nowadays those of us who want contraception can get it easily, and it's simple to use, although all methods require you to plan ahead. Some religions don't allow birth control, as they believe people should only have sex to produce a baby. That's fine if you're happy to wait to have sex until you're married and ready to start a family. But unfortunately, often couples who aren't using contraception for whatever reason don't abstain from sex—they go ahead and convince themselves they won't get pregnant or that one of the old wives' tales will work for them.

Not so. Contraception, used properly, is the only way to prevent a pregnancy. And teenage girls are very fertile and get pregnant more easily than older women. The United States has the highest teen pregnancy rate of all developed countries. More than one million teens get pregnant each year. Very few of those girls will have actually planned for and wanted a baby, so that adds up to an awful lot of misery.

Where to Go for Contraception

This is a general guide—"Methods of Contraception" and "Emergency Contraception" (pages 129–155) give more details about where you can get each kind. The advice you get at health centers and doctors' offices is confidential, which means the doctor or nurse won't tell anyone that you visited or what you saw them for. You can go to:

- your family doctor;
- a health center;
- a gynecologist.

Call Planned Parenthood at 1-800-230-PLAN to find your nearest clinic, or visit their Web site at http://www.plannedparenthood.org. They'll also send you free pamphlets on all the methods of contraception.

To find out what happens when you go to your family doctor or a health center for contraceptive advice, see "Doctors and Other Health Professionals" in chapter 13.

Myths About Preventing Pregnancy

Preventing pregnancy is straightforward. Any method that doesn't involve contraception won't work. Here are some common myths.

You can't get pregnant . . .
- *if the girl doesn't orgasm.* Yes, you can;
- *if the girl hasn't started her period.* Yes, you can. A girl can ovulate (release her monthly egg) before her first period;
- *the first time you have sex.* 'Fraid so;
- *if you have sex standing up.* Yes, you can;
- *if the girl jumps up and down after sex.* Nonsense;
- *during your period.* Yes, you can. Some girls ovulate during their period. Also, sperm can live for up to five days, so they could be still be hanging around if she ovulates soon after her period;
- *if the boy puts his penis in, but takes it out again quickly, or pulls out before he comes.* Yes, you can. Long before a boy comes, his penis leaks a clear liquid called pre-ejaculate that contains thousands of sperm. That means as soon as the penis is erect there may be sperm on the tip. Many teenagers get pregnant each

year because pulling out, or "withdrawal," is their
only method of preventing pregnancy;

• *if you wash your vagina out with cola, lemon juice, or
other liquid after sex.* Sperm swim much too fast to be
flushed out, so this doesn't work either. Plus you
should never flood your vagina and cervix with liquids
of any kind, as it disturbs the natural balance of the
bacteria there.

Natural Method

One idea that contains *some* truth is that there's a safe period
when the girl can't get pregnant. But this "natural" family
planning method is only used by couples who are content to
have a baby anyway, because it takes a lot of commitment by
both partners to stick to the guidelines and only have sex at
certain times. You need special charts to record the girl's
temperature and other bodily signs ("fertility indicators") each
day over six months to work out when you might be able to
have sex without her getting pregnant. After that she has to
monitor her fertility indicators on a daily basis. This is a very
complicated method and the failure rate is high. As such, it's not
for couples who definitely don't want a baby, and of course it
offers no protection against STDs.

METHODS OF CONTRACEPTION

The only way to be 100 percent sure you won't get pregnant is not to have any sexual contact. But if you are going to have sex, make sure you are totally clued in when it comes to contraception.

Here we'll go through the various options available for protection against pregnancy. Contraception aims to prevent conception, which is when the male sperm joins with the female egg inside her body and grows into a baby.

The vital thing to remember is that **only condoms protect against STDs as well as pregnancy** because they form a barrier between your vagina and your partner's penis and keep the secretions separate. Therefore, whichever other contraceptive method you use, you should always use condoms as well to avoid infections. However, if you're in a long-term relationship and both of you have been tested for STDs—and have been given the all clear—you could stop using condoms in addition to another form of contraception. But bear in mind that, for either of you, any sexual contact outside the relationship puts you at risk of catching STDs and infecting your regular partner.

Using a condom for sex is known as safer sex. Note this isn't SAFE sex—there's no such thing, because all sex carries a risk of pregnancy or catching an STD, however careful you are and whatever contraceptive method you use. The only way to be 100 percent safe is not to have sex at all!

It may seem annoying, but at present, all contraception— apart from male condoms—are used by the girl. This leads some people to believe that contraception is the girl's responsibility. And because it's the girl who'll literally end up holding the baby if she gets pregnant, this makes some boys even more casual about contraception. Boys with this attitude are to be avoided.

All the hormonal methods (both kinds of contraceptive pill, injections, implants, the IUS, the patch, and the emergency pill) alter your hormonal balance and have different potential risks and side effects, and they're not all suitable for everyone. If you're interested in using one of these methods, the doctor or nurse you see for contraceptive advice will take your medical history and talk to you about which would suit you best. That's why it's a bad idea to lend or borrow pills or other contraceptive methods—they can make you very ill if they weren't prescribed for you.

Please be aware that this is only a general guide to contraception, and should not be relied upon as a substitute for medical advice.

If the method of contraception you choose doesn't suit you, don't just stop using it. Some couples try a few different kinds before they hit on the one they like best.

In order, this chapter will look at the pros and cons of:

- male and female condoms
- combination pill
- progestin-only pill
- contraceptive injections
- diaphragms and caps plus spermicide
- intrauterine devices (IUS and IUD)
- contraceptive patch
- the last resort: emergency contraception

Condoms

What Are They and How Do They Work?

There are two types: the *male condom*, which is what most people use, and the *female condom*. Made of very thin rubber (latex) or soft plastic (polyurethane), the male condom fits over the boy's erect penis. The female condom, also made of soft plastic, is bigger, a bit like a small bag, and is used to line the vagina. When the boy ejaculates, his sperm is caught inside the condom.

How Effective Are Condoms at Preventing Pregnancy?

Male Condom

If used according to the instructions it's 98 percent effective, which means two women out of every hundred who use them properly will get pregnant. Less careful use means more women will become pregnant.

Female Condom

If used according to instructions it's 95 percent effective.

What Makes Condoms Less Effective at Preventing Pregnancy?

Male Condom

* It can split or burst.
* The boy's penis can touch the girl's vagina before the condom goes on.
* It can slip off.

Female Condom

* The boy's penis can slip around the side of it on entry.
* It can fall out.

Both

* They may not have been put on/in properly.
* They can be damaged by sharp nails or jewelry.

Advantages

* They protect both partners against some STDs as well as preventing pregnancy.
* There are no side effects (unless you're allergic to latex rubber or spermicide).
* You only need to use them when you want to have sex.
* They're easy to buy (male condoms, anyway).
* The female condom can go in anytime before sex.
* The female condom is good for boys who lose their erection in a male condom.
* Male condoms come in different shapes and sizes, so there's a type to suit any boy.

Disadvantages

* Rarely, some people are allergic to latex rubber and/or the spermicide that comes with the condom (spermicide is a chemical that kills sperm—see page 146 for more information). Polyurethane (nonlatex condoms) aren't lubricated with spermicide, so ask your pharmacist or someone at a family-planning clinic about using this kind.
* Putting on the male condom interrupts sex.
* Some boys lose their erection once they put a condom on.
* They can be tricky to get on/in and keep on/in if you're not used to them, so it's best to practice before you have sex rather than waiting until you're in the middle of a steamy situation. (You can do this on your own! Sounds

crazy, but try the male condom on a banana.)
* Not all clinics stock female condoms and they're more expensive to buy than male condoms.

Using Condoms

All packets contain instructions, so read these carefully. You can also ask the doctor or nurse you see for contraceptive services for advice. Store condoms in a cool, dry place. Only keep them in a wallet or bag temporarily, and make sure the packet doesn't get bent, as it might weaken the condom. Check the expiration date on the packet (old condoms can rot!), and use a new condom each time you have sex. Take the condom out of the packet carefully, keeping sharp nails and jewelry away.

Male Condom

* At the closed end, you'll find a reservoir, which catches the sperm during sex. Squeeze this between your finger and thumb to get rid of any air. This also shows that you've got the condom the right way to roll onto the boy's penis.
* It's vital to put the condom onto the boy's penis as soon as it becomes erect and before it touches the girl's genital area. Hold the reservoir end and roll it all the way down the penis.
* If it won't roll down, it's inside out. Throw it away and take out a fresh one because it may have sperm on it that would end up inside the girl once it's turned the right way. Don't use it!

" SAFE "
BANANA

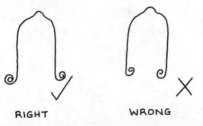

RIGHT   WRONG

* Once the boy has come and while the penis is still hard, he should hold the condom firmly around the base of his penis while he pulls out of the girl's vagina. This is so no semen is spilled and so that the condom doesn't stay inside her.
* Wrap up the condom and trash it. Don't put it in the toilet—our sewage system can't process them, and they'll end up on beaches along with all the tampons people can't be bothered to dispose of properly.

Female Condom

* Put it in before the penis touches the girl's genitals. It can go in any time before sex, though.
* To insert the condom, you can lie down, squat, or put one leg up on a chair, whichever is most comfortable.
* The female condom is like a bag with a rubber ring at the closed end, plus one around the open end like the male condom. Squeeze the inner ring between your thumb and middle finger. Keep your index finger (the one you use to point) in the center of this ring to hold it steady.
* Spread your vaginal lips with your other hand, then push the squeezed ring as far into your vagina as you can.
* Then put a finger inside the condom and push the inner ring as far back as it will go.
* The outer ring should be hanging outside your vagina, up against the outside.
* It's best for you or your partner to guide the penis in to make sure it doesn't slip down the side. The female condom fits loosely and will move about during sex.

* To remove, twist the outer ring closed to keep in the semen, then pull the condom out. Wrap it and trash it.

Where Can I Get Condoms?

Condoms are available at very low cost at some health clinics such as Planned Parenthood. You can buy them cheaply at pharmacies, gas stations, and supermarkets, and there are often vending machines in public restrooms. There are lots of different types of male condoms—for example, ones with ribbing that are supposed to increase sensation, or extra-thin ones that claim to feel more natural.

You can also buy female condoms at health clinics or pharmacies.

Any Other Considerations?

* Sexual-health experts recommend using male condoms for oral sex on boys to prevent passing on STDs. You'd probably want to use condoms without spermicide for this, although spermicide won't harm you if swallowed.
* Some people like to use lubrication to help the penis slip in more easily. All condoms are lubricated, some male ones with spermicide (see page 146 for more on spermicide). You can use extra spermicide if you want to be even safer and/or want more lubrication. Regarding nonspermicidal lubricants, go for water-based ones such as K-Y liquid or jelly, available from supermarkets and pharmacies. Don't use oil-based lubricants, such as body oils, petroleum jelly (Vaseline), creams, or lotions, because they'll break down some types of condoms in a few minutes, leaving holes.

Combination Pill

What Is It and How Does It Work?

It's normally just called the Pill, but there are several different brand names. All contain man-made versions of two female hormones, estrogen and progesterone.

Its main action is to stop your ovaries from releasing an egg, which, if fertilized by a boy's sperm, grows into a baby. If you haven't released an egg, you can't possibly get pregnant. In addition, it thickens the mucus at the entrance of your cervix (neck of the womb), which makes it harder for a sperm to get through in search of an egg. Plus it thins your womb lining, making it less likely that an egg, if fertilized, could implant there and grow into a baby.

How Effective Is the Combination Pill at Preventing Pregnancy?

Taken according to the instructions, the combination pill is over 99 percent effective, which means that on average and when taken properly, less than one woman in a hundred will get pregnant in a year if she's having regular sex. With less careful use, more women will become pregnant. And the combination pill does not protect against STDs, so it should always be used in combination with a condom.

What Makes the Combination Pill Less Effective at Preventing Pregnancy?

* Missing one or more pills. Refer to the pill packet leaflet, but the general advice is as follows: *If you're LESS than twelve hours late*, take your missed pill immediately and the rest of the pack as normal. You're still covered by the Pill, so you don't need extra contraception. *If you're MORE than*

twelve hours late, take your last missed pill now but leave any others you've forgotten. It is very important to use a condom as well for the next seven days. Read the pill packet leaflet, contact your doctor, or call Planned Parenthood at 1-800-230-PLAN for advice, as different brands of pill require different action depending on how many pills are left in the packet.

* Starting a new pack late.
* Throwing up within three hours of taking a pill or if you have very severe diarrhea for twenty-four hours or more. Keep taking your pills but use another form of contraception as well, such as the condom, while you're ill and for seven days after you get better.
* Some prescribed medicines, such as antibiotics, can interfere with the working of your pill, so find out if you have to use a condom also while you're taking the medicine and for seven days afterward.

Advantages

* You usually have shorter, lighter, less painful periods.
* It doesn't interfere with sex.
* It can reduce PMS symptoms.
* It protects against some pelvic infections and ovarian and uterine cancer.
* Many women find that the combined pill improves skin problems. In fact, some doctors prescribe a combination pill, like Ortho Tri-cyclen to treat acne. Your doctor can advise you on whether this treatment is right for you.

Disadvantages

* You have to remember to take it every day.

* Temporary side effects that should stop within the first three months can include: feeling nauseous, losing or gaining weight, headaches, sore boobs, moodiness, and bleeding between periods. If side effects continue for more than three months, talk to your doctor. A change of pill may help.

* The Pill doesn't protect against STDs, so it's important to use condoms as well if you think you might be at risk.

* Rare but serious side effects include increased risks of blood clots in veins or arteries (this risk is further increased in smokers), breast cancer, and cervical cancer.

* Medical conditions that mean you can't take the combination pill include severe migraines, high blood pressure, and unexplained vaginal bleeding (e.g., between periods or after sex).

Taking the Combination Pill

There isn't space here to go into each different type of combination pill in detail, so make sure you understand what the doctor who prescribes yours says, and read the packet pamphlet in full. If you have questions, go back to the doctor or call the Planned Parenthood help line at 1-800-230-PLAN.

There are two main types: either you take one a day for twenty-one days and then have a seven-day break, when your period comes, or you have what are known as "combination pills" and you take one a day for twenty-eight days, even during your period. With some pills, you're protected from pregnancy from the day you take the first pill. With others, you're not protected until day seven or even day fifteen.

Try to get into a routine of taking your pill at approximately the same time each day, for example, after you've brushed your teeth each morning. Because you need to use condoms as well for the next seven days if you take your pill more than twelve hours late (see pages 136–137), you need to get a sense of your regular pill-taking time so you know if you're late taking it.

Where Can I Get the Combination Pill?
It has to be prescribed by a doctor or nurse, so you can get it from your gynecologist, your family doctor, or a health clinic.

Progestin-Only Pill (POP or Mini-Pill)

What Is It and How Does It Work?
It contains man-made progesterone (called progestin), and works by thickening the mucus at your womb entrance to stop sperm from getting through. It also thins your womb lining and may stop the release of your monthly egg. The progestin-only pill is slightly less reliable than the combination pill, and the fact that you have to take it at exactly the same time each day is a problem for some women. Like the combination pill, the mini-pill doesn't protect against STDs and should always be used in combination with condoms.

How Effective Is the Progestin-Only Pill at Preventing Pregnancy?
If a person follows the instructions, the progestin-only pill is 99 percent effective (one user in every hundred will get pregnant per year). There will be more pregnancies among less careful users.

What Makes the Progestin-Only Pill Less Effective at Preventing Pregnancy?

If you miss a pill and *if you're LESS than three hours late*, take your missed pill now and the next at the usual time, even if it means taking two pills in one day. You're still covered by the pill, so you don't need extra contraception. *If you're MORE than three hours late*, take your missed pill now and the next at the usual time, even if it means taking two pills in one day. Use a condom as well for the next seven days.

Advantages

* It doesn't have serious side effects, such as an increased risk of thrombosis, like the combination pill. This means it's safer for smokers.
* It doesn't interfere with sex.
* It may reduce PMS and make periods lighter and less painful.
* It can be used by those who can't take estrogen, which the combination pill contains.

Disadvantages

* It must be taken at the same time each day or it doesn't work. It's not often prescribed to teenagers for this reason.
* Your periods may not come regularly. They might stop or come more often. This might settle down, but you may start to worry that you're pregnant. A different progestin-only pill may help with this.
* Some women get acne or sore boobs for the first few months.
* Small fluid-filled cysts may appear on your ovaries. They'll usually go away without treatment and most

girls don't know they've got them, but some find they cause pelvic pain.

* It offers no protection against STDs, so use a condom as well.
* Medical conditions that mean you can't take the mini-pill include liver disease, having had a heart attack, and unexplained vaginal bleeding (e.g., between periods or after sex).

Taking the Progestin-Only Pill

You take the first one on the first day of your period and are protected from pregnancy immediately. A pill is taken at the same time each day, every day. When you finish one pack, you start the next immediately, so that you're taking pills all through your period.

Where Can I Get the Progestin-Only Pill?

Anywhere you can get the combination pill.

Contraceptive Injections

What Are They and How Do They Work?

There are two types of contraceptive injection: Depo-Provera, the most common, and Lunelle, which is newer and used less frequently. Depo-Provera protects you from pregnancy for twelve weeks, Lunelle for one month. Both work by stopping the release of your monthly egg, thinning your womb lining, and thickening the mucus at the entrance to your womb. Both contain a man-made version of the hormone progesterone. Lunelle also contains estrogen, as in a combination pill. They don't protect against STDs, so condoms should be used as well.

How Effective Are Contraceptive Injections at Preventing Pregnancy?

Over 99 percent.

What Makes Contraceptive Injections Less Effective at Preventing Pregnancy?

Not getting your next injection on time or taking medicine that interferes with the injection. Medicines you buy over the counter at the pharmacy won't affect it, but some prescribed ones may (this doesn't include antibiotics). Ask the doctor who gives you your injections for a list of medications.

Advantages

* There are no serious health risks for Depo-Provera because the injections don't contain estrogen, so they're suitable for smokers.
* They don't interfere with sex.
* You don't have to think about contraception for the duration of the injection.
* The injection isn't absorbed by the stomach like the pill, so its effectiveness isn't affected by vomiting and diarrhea.
* They give some protection against uterine cancer and pelvic inflammatory disease (PID).
* Depo-Provera can be used by girls who can't take estrogen, which is in the combination pill.

Disadvantages

* Most people's periods change. They can be irregular and longer than usual, may stop completely, or you may bleed often, though your periods will be light. You might bleed

irregularly for a few months after if you stop the injections.

* Possible side effects include weight gain, headaches, acne, sore boobs, mood swings, and bloating.

* As the injection works for four or twelve weeks, it can't be removed from your body, so if you get side effects, they may go on for as long as the injection lasts and for some time afterward. Lunelle works for a shorter time, so if you experience side effects, you can stop using it sooner.

* Your periods and fertility (ability to conceive a baby) can take up to a year to return to normal after you've stopped the injections.

* Injections don't protect against STDs, so you still need to use condoms.

* Medical conditions that mean you can't have the contraceptive injection are the same as for the mini-pill.

Using Contraceptive Injections

The hormone is injected into a muscle, usually in your bottom. You can get the injection any time from the first day of your period to the fifth day and be protected against pregnancy immediately.

Where Can I Get a Contraceptive Injection?

It has to be given by a nurse or doctor.

Any Other Considerations?

Contraceptive injections aren't suitable if you've had severe depression or if you don't want your periods to change.

Diaphragms and Caps

What Are They and How Do They Work?

Diaphragms (pronounced *die-a-frams*) and caps are inserted into your vagina and fitted over your cervix (neck of the womb) to prevent sperm entering your womb. They're always used along with spermicide, a chemical jelly or foam that kills sperm. Diaphragms are circular domes made of thin rubber with a flexible rim. Caps are smaller.

How Effective Are Diaphragms and Caps at Preventing Pregnancy?

Between 92 and 96 percent effective if used according to the instructions. That's between four and eight women getting pregnant for every hundred women using a cap or diaphragm as a contraceptive. Less careful use means more pregnancies.

What Makes the Diaphragm or Cap Less Effective at Preventing Pregnancy?

* Not having it fitted properly over your cervix.
* Using it without spermicide.
* Having sex three hours or more after putting it in and not using extra spermicide.
* Having sex a second time with your cap or diaphragm in and not using extra spermicide.
* Taking out your cap or diaphragm less than six hours after you had sex.
* Using oil-based products with your cap or diaphragm (they can weaken the rubber).

Advantages

* You only use it when you have sex.
* It has no associated health risks.
* It may protect against cervical cancer and some STDs.
* You can put it in any time before sex (but reach up your vagina and put extra spermicide around the cap or diaphragm if it's been in more than three hours).

Disadvantages

* Putting it in can interrupt sex.
* Spermicide can be messy and feel wet to you and your partner.
* You have to remember to add more spermicide around your cap or diaphragm each time you have sex.
* It takes a while to learn how to put a cap or diaphragm in easily.
* Some diaphragm users get frequent bouts of cystitis (see page 175), but changing to a cap might help.

Using the Diaphragm or Cap

The doctor or nurse who examines you will tell you whether a cap or diaphragm is most suitable, find one in your size, and show you how to put it in. The method of insertion is slightly different with each but involves putting spermicide cream or jelly on the cap or diaphragm, compressing the springy rim between your fingers, and pushing it high into your vagina to cover your cervix. Whichever you use, it has to be kept in for at least six hours after you last had sex, but no more than thirty hours for the diaphragm and forty-eight hours for the cap. Then you wash and dry it and store it in its box.

Where Can I Get a Diaphragm or Cap?

A family-planning clinic or your doctor. They'll give you a practice cap or diaphragm in your size to try at home, but you mustn't rely on this for contraception. Wear it when you go back so they can check that you've put it in properly, then they'll give you one to use for contraception.

Any Other Considerations?

You can use a cap or diaphragm during your period when you have sex, as it will collect the blood. If you gain or lose more than seven pounds, talk to whoever prescribed your cap or diaphragm, as you might need a different size.

Spermicides: A Note

This sperm-killing chemical comes in several forms, such as jellies, foams, and creams, and many condoms are lubricated with it. Spermicides are used with diaphragms and caps for extra peace of mind. When choosing a spermicide, it's important to go for one containing Nonoxynol-9, because that can also kill the HIV virus, which causes AIDS, and some other STD germs. Spermicides sometimes cause irritation, but a change of brand should help. Ask your doctor, nurse, or pharmacist for advice. Never use spermicide as your only form of contraception, as it can't prevent pregnancy on its own.

You can buy spermicides from pharmacies and health clinics.

Intrauterine Devices

What Are They and How Do They Work?

There are two types: the IUS (intrauterine system), which is a small, flat T-shaped plastic device that contains the hormone progestin; and the IUD (intrauterine device), which comes in several shapes, and is made of copper and plastic. Both kinds are fitted into your womb and have one or two threads that hang from the neck of your womb (these are so you can check that it's still in place).

The IUS works a bit like the mini-pill in that the hormone thickens the mucus from your cervix, making it harder for sperm to swim through; it thins your womb lining, and you may stop releasing eggs.

The IUD contains no hormones. It prevents sperm from reaching the egg, but, if an egg does become fertilized, the IUD will then prevent it from settling in the womb. This used to be known as the coil. The IUD and IUS don't protect against STDs, so you need to use condoms as well.

How Effective Are Intrauterine Devices at Preventing Pregnancy?

The IUS is over 99 percent effective, which means that out of every hundred women who use it, less then one will get pregnant per year. With the IUD, one per hundred will get pregnant.

What Makes Them Less Effective at Preventing Pregnancy?

Nothing (including antibiotics) interferes with the IUS or IUD as long as they stay in place.

Advantages

* Like the progestin-only pill, there are no serious health risks associated with the IUS. Also, the hormone isn't absorbed by the stomach like the Pill, so its effectiveness isn't affected by vomiting and diarrhea.
* The IUS works for five years, the IUD for between three

and ten, depending on which kind you have.

* They don't interfere with sex.

* An IUS usually gets rid of period pain and makes your periods shorter and lighter after three months.

Disadvantages

* With the IUS, it's usual to have some irregular bleeding between periods for the first three months. You also might get headaches, acne, and sore boobs in that time. Some women also get fluid-filled cysts on their ovaries that usually disappear on their own. Medical conditions that mean you can't have the IUS include liver disease, untreated STDs, and unexplained vaginal bleeding.

* With the IUD, periods may be longer, heavier, or more painful for the first few months. It's also easier to develop a pelvic infection from an STD.

* With the IUD and the IUS, your womb can push it out or it can move, so go back to the doctor or nurse who put it in for you if you think this has happened. They'll also teach you to check the hanging threads each month to make sure the device is in place. You can still use tampons, though.

* Rarely, both the IUD and IUS can pierce your womb or cervix when fitted and will have to be surgically removed.

* They don't protect against STDs, so condoms should be used as well.

Using the IUD or IUS

They're fitted toward the end of or just after your period. The doctor or nurse will examine you inside to find the size and position of your womb, and they'll talk to you about whether to have a painkiller or local anesthetic before the device is put in. Period-type pain and a bit of bleeding is common for a few days after fitting. An IUD works as soon as it's put in. An IUS works immediately if it goes in within the first seven days of your menstrual cycle. The doctor or nurse will show you how to feel for the strings at the top of your vagina once a month to check that the device is still in position.

Where Can I Get the IUD or IUS?
Health clinics, some family doctors, and gynecologists.

The Contraceptive Patch

What Is It and How Does It Work?
The Ortho Evra patch is a thin, beige patch two inches by two inches in size that you stick on your skin. It releases two hormones, estrogen and progestin, and works in a similar way to the combination pill. The patch stops the release of your monthly egg, while thickening your cervical mucus and making the womb lining thinner. It doesn't protect against STDs, so you'll need to use condoms as well.

How Effective Is the Contraceptive Patch at Preventing Pregnancy?
Over 99 percent.

What Makes the Contraceptive Patch Less Effective at Preventing Pregnancy?
* Some prescribed medicines, including certain antibiotics and epilepsy drugs. Check with your doctor before taking any medication.
* If it falls off and isn't put back immediately.
* Forgetting to put on a new patch when you're supposed to (see "Using the Contraceptive Patch").

Advantages

* It doesn't interrupt sex.
* It's easy to use.
* It generally makes periods lighter and less painful.
* It isn't absorbed by the stomach like the Pill, so its effectiveness isn't affected by vomiting and diarrhea.
* You only have to think about it once a week, at patch-change time.

Disadvantages

* People might see or feel it, depending on where it is.
* It can irritate the skin.
* It doesn't protect against STDs, so you need condoms as well.
* Side effects can include headaches, feeling sick, sore boobs, mood swings, and weight gain or loss. They should stop after a few months.
* Bleeding between periods in the first few months is common.
* There's a very low risk of serious side effects, the same as with the combination pill. They include blood clots and an increased risk of breast cancer.
* Medical conditions that mean you can't have the patch include severe migraines, high blood pressure, and unexplained vaginal bleeding.

Using the Contraceptive Patch

On the first day of your period, you put on a patch. They're very sticky and can go on any body area as long as it's not hairy. Upper arm, bottom, and abdomen are popular sites. You take it off after seven days and put on a new one. After three weeks you have a patch-free week, when your period will come. On day eight of your patch-free time, you apply another patch, whether or not you're still bleeding, and the cycle begins again.

Where Can I Get the Contraceptive Patch?
Family-planning doctors, sexual-health clinics, and most family doctors and gynecologists.

Any Other Considerations?
If you forget to put another patch on at the end of your patch-free week and more than forty-eight hours have gone by from when you should have done so, put on a patch as soon as you remember and use condoms for the next seven days. You can't decorate the patch or use body creams on it, as it might come off or its effectiveness may be reduced. It should stay on through a bath or shower, but if it slips off and is still sticky, slap it back on. Soap won't affect it, but dry the patch well after it's been wet. If it's been off for more than twenty-four hours, you'll need to use condoms for the next seven days.

EMERGENCY CONTRACEPTION

What Is Emergency Contraception?

It's for use if your usual contraception fails—for example, if your condom splits or you've forgotten to take some of your contraceptive pills, or if you've had unprotected sex—to prevent you from becoming pregnant.

There are two methods: taking emergency pills and having an IUD (intrauterine device) fitted in your womb.

Emergency contraception works by stopping the release of an egg or, if an egg has been fertilized, stopping it from settling into the wall of your womb. Medical and legal experts agree that emergency contraception prevents pregnancy; it doesn't cause an abortion. An abortion can only take place if a fertilized egg that's implanted in the wall of the womb is removed.

Method One: Emergency Contraceptive Pills

What Are They and How Do They Work?

These used to be known as the "morning-after pill," but are no longer called that because it's misleading. They can be taken up to three days (seventy-two hours) after unprotected sex, but the sooner they're taken, the more effective they are. That's why if you think you've been at risk, it's important to seek help as soon as you can.

Emergency contraceptive pills contain the hormone progestin, and they come in packs of one or two pills. The pill or pills work by stopping your body from releasing an egg or, if an egg has already been fertilized by a boy's sperm, stopping it from settling into the wall of your womb, where it would start to grow into a baby.

How Effective Are Emergency Contraceptive Pills at Preventing Pregnancy?

They work very well but are more effective the sooner they're taken after unprotected sex. If taken within twenty-four hours after unprotected sex, ninety-five out of a hundred potential pregnancies will be prevented. If taken seventy-two hours after unprotected sex, fifty-eight out of a hundred potential pregnancies will be prevented.

What Makes Emergency Contraceptive Pills Less Effective at Preventing Pregnancy?

* Throwing up within two hours of taking the pill or pills. If this happens, talk to whomever gave it or them to you. They may give you more or suggest you have an IUD fitted.

* Taking the pill or pills more than seventy-two hours after unprotected sex.

* Not taking the pill or pills according to the instructions.

* Having had unprotected sex either since your last period (i.e., before the session of unprotected sex you got the pill or pills for) or after taking the emergency pill.

Advantages

* If you've had unprotected sex or your contraception failed, taking emergency contraception pills according to the instructions will make it very unlikely that you'll become pregnant.

* Emergency pills don't carry any long-term or serious health risks.

* Almost anyone can use emergency pills, but tell the doctor, nurse, or pharmacist who's giving them to you if you're taking any medicines or have any illnesses to make sure it's OK for you to take the pills.

Disadvantages

* You'll still have to wait for your period to find out whether you're pregnant or not.

* There can be the following side effects: headaches, feeling nauseous (one in four users) and, with a few girls (six in a hundred), actually throwing up, abdominal pain, dizziness, and sore boobs.

Using Emergency Contraceptive Pills

You take the pill (if there are two in your pack, you take them together) as soon as possible, within seventy-two hours after unprotected sex. Your period might come earlier than usual or up to a week late, but it will generally be within a few days of its usual time. Some girls get breakthrough bleeding before their next period, which can vary from a tiny bit of blood (spotting) to a lot.

You don't need to see a doctor or nurse once you've taken emergency contraceptive pills unless

- your period's more than seven days late or it's shorter or lighter than usual (you could be pregnant);
- you get sudden abdominal pain and haven't yet had a normal period (this can be a rare, serious condition called an ectopic pregnancy, where a baby starts to grow outside the womb);
- you think you've caught an STD.

Where Can I Get Emergency Contraceptive Pills?

From family doctors, health clinics, gynecologists, some emergency rooms (call to check before you go), and some pharmacies. A few school nurses also offer it.

If you need emergency pills in the evening or over the weekend, try a twenty-four-hour pharmacy or a hospital emergency room. To find a Planned Parenthood affiliated health center near you, call 1-800-230-PLAN.

Any Other Considerations?

* One dose of emergency pill is designed to protect against pregnancy from one session of unprotected sex. So if you have unprotected sex again before your next period,

you're not protected by the emergency pills and need to use another form of contraception.

* If you do end up using emergency contraception, you'd be wise to go and discuss your usual method of contraception and perhaps switch to something more reliable or easier for you to keep up. If you weren't using any contraception, now's the time to remedy the situation so you don't have to go through this again.

* Emergency pills are not meant for regular use. It's essential to use contraception each time you have sex.

Method Two: IUD

The IUD can be fitted in your womb up to five days after unprotected sex, and it works by either stopping an egg from being fertilized by sperm or stopping a fertilized egg from implanting in the womb. It's very effective (nearly 100 percent) at preventing pregnancy provided it's fitted within the five-day time frame. You go back to the doctor or nurse who fitted it three to four weeks later, whether you've had your period or not, to make sure you're not pregnant. The IUD can either be removed after your period has arrived or kept in as a regular method of contraception.

Any Other Considerations?
Most women can use the IUD for emergency contraception, but it's best to call the clinic or hospital beforehand to make sure there's someone there trained to fit one. Try a family-planning clinic, health clinic, or hospital emergency room. Some family doctors and most gynecologists also fit them.

CHAPTER ELEVEN

Sexually Transmitted Diseases and Women's Health

Ideally, everyone's sexual experiences should be happy, healthy ones, but sadly sexually transmitted diseases (STDs) are on the rise among teenagers. One out of every four teens in the United States will be infected by an STD. But this could be the tip of the iceberg because many STDs don't show symptoms, and if you don't know you're sick, you won't seek help. That's why it's vital to learn how to take care of your sexual health so you can protect yourself and your partner from disease.

You can't tell someone has an STD by looking at them. Because so many STDs don't show symptoms, a person may have a disease that they can pass on to you without knowing it, or vice versa. The best advice is to always use condoms and, with a new partner, for both of you to get tested at a clinic before anything sexual happens, to make sure nothing will be passed between you.

Guilt and embarrassment stop us from seeking an expert opinion if we're worried something's wrong down below. But doctors and nurses see people's bodies all day and are not even remotely shocked by your nakedness. Clinic staff are skilled at doing their job in a friendly but professional manner and aren't going to give you a sidelong "I know what you've been up to—whatever you've caught, it serves you right for having sex!"

look. Honestly! Remember that your visit and everything you tell health professionals is confidential, which means they can't pass on your details. (For more on confidentiality, see page 207.)

This chapter is all about STDs. Related to this is the health of your reproductive system (genitals and internal parts such as your womb and cervix), as some infections in this area that aren't sexually transmitted *as such*, can nonetheless be passed on via sex. Toward the end of the chapter you'll find information on infections that mainly affect women.

In this chapter you'll find:

- Virgins Can Have STDs Too; STDs: General Symptoms; If You Think You Have an STD
- STDs—What's What: Chlamydia; Genital Herpes; Genital Warts; Gonorrhea; Hepatitis B; HIV and AIDS; Non-Specific Genital Infections (NSGIs); Pubic Lice (Crabs); Scabies; Syphilis; Trichomonas Vaginalis (TV)
- Women's Health: Bacterial Vaginosis (BV); Cystitis; Pelvic Inflammatory Disease (PID); Yeast Infections (Thrush)

Virgins Can Have STDs Too

I'm often asked if virgins can have STDs. The answer is yes— you don't have to have full sex to catch an STD. If a virgin has had any sexual contact at all with another person, that is, if they've touched a partner's genitals or if a partner handled their own genitals and then touched yours, germs can be passed on. Genital warts can be carried on fingers, and herpes can be spread through oral sex. So if you or your partner have been intimate with another person, it would be wise to get tested before having any sexual contact with each other. Visiting a clinic together shows you both take each other's health and well-being seriously—and that's sexy! You won't be seen by the doctor together, by the way.

If you go for a general checkup at a clinic, you're routinely tested for chlamydia, gonorrhea, trichomonas vaginalis, and syphilis. You'll also be asked what type of sex (e.g., penetrative sex or oral sex) you've been having and with whom, and if you have any symptoms to see if you need further tests. It's important to be honest with the doctor or nurse so you get tested for all infections you might have come into contact with.

STDs: General Symptoms

Although you may have no symptoms with an STD—and girls are even less likely to show symptoms than boys—for both sexes, things to look out for are

- pain or burning when peeing;
- sore genitals;
- pain during sex;
- peeing more often than usual;
- an unusual discharge from the vagina or penis, perhaps smelly, thick, yellow, white, or cloudy;
- rashes, itching, blisters, sores, or lumps on or near the genitals;
- for girls, bleeding after sex or between periods.

It's a good idea to get to know what your genitals look like and the consistency and smell of your usual secretions (see chapter

1 for more information on this). That way, it'll be easier to spot if something's wrong.

If you've had any of the above symptoms but they've stopped, seek help anyway, because if you do have an STD, it will still be lurking. STDs don't go away on their own—they need treatment. Most can be easily cured, but the earlier they're treated, the simpler they are to zap. As long as you have an STD you can pass it on, and they can cause a lot of damage to the reproductive system, particularly in girls. If untreated, some STDs can make it hard to have a baby in the future. Sometimes girls are left infertile, which means they can't have a baby at all.

If You Think You Have an STD

* Don't have sex or sexual contact until you've been diagnosed and your treatment's finished.

* Your partner needs to be tested and possibly treated too, otherwise you'll pass the infection back and forth between you. If you want, the clinic staff will help you think about how to talk to him or her about this.

* Your previous partners, if any, should also be contacted and urged to get a checkup. Clinics recognize that this can be horribly embarrassing, so some have "contact slips" that you can put previous partners' details on and then you or the clinic will send them out. The slip says that the person may have been exposed to an STD and suggests they get checked out. It doesn't mention your name or what the disease may be, so your confidentiality is protected.

STDs: WHAT'S WHAT

There are over twenty-five STDs, but here we'll look at some of the more common ones. If you think you might have an infection, there's only one way to find out for sure: visit a doctor's office or a clinic. Staff are happy to do checkups, so don't worry that you're wasting anyone's time.

To find out what happens when you go to your family doctor or a clinic for help with STDs, see "Doctors and Other Health Professionals" in chapter 13.

Chlamydia

Chlamydia is caused by bacteria. Found in semen and vaginal fluid, chlamydia is very common in teenagers and is generally passed on during sex, including oral sex. If chlamydia isn't treated, it can cause serious health problems. It doesn't cause cervical cancer, as some people think, but can lead to pelvic inflammatory disease (PID) in girls, which can cause long-term abdominal pain, permanently blocked Fallopian tubes, and infertility. It is the most common, and invisible, STD in the United States.

Symptoms
Nearly 70 percent of females and 50 percent of males show no symptoms, so many cases remain undiagnosed. However, one to three weeks or even several months after infection you may notice the following symptoms:

Girls: unusual vaginal discharge; pain when peeing;

bleeding between periods; lower abdominal pain; bleeding after or during sex; pain during sex.

Boys: a cloudy, white, watery discharge from the penis; pain when peeing; sore, swollen testicles.

Tests and Treatments
A doctor or nurse will take a swab from the areas that may be infected and may ask for a urine sample. Treatment is with antibiotics.

Protecting Against Chlamydia
Use condoms whenever you have sex, including oral sex. Latex squares, available from health clinics and pharmacies, should be used for oral sex on a girl.

Genital Herpes

There are two types of cold sore viruses: herpes simplex 1 and herpes simplex 2. Most cases of genital herpes used to be caused by herpes simplex 2, while herpes simplex 1 was responsible for facial sores. But because oral sex is now more widely practiced, the two types of virus have been swapping sites, so facial or genital herpes can be either type 1 or type 2. (The fingers are the third most usual area for herpes simplex sores, known as *whitlows*, because fingers often have cuts, which allows the virus to enter the skin.) Most people who have the virus only have one type. However, you can catch the type you don't have from someone else. That means you could end up with one type on your face and the other on your genitals. Type 1 and type 2 look similar, so you can only find out which one you've caught by having a blood test. You can catch genital herpes by (1) having sexual intercourse with someone who has genital herpes, (2) being given oral sex by someone with facial herpes (cold sores), or (3) being touched around the genitals by a person with herpes (whitlows) on their fingers. You can't spread the virus to other parts of your own body, and it will only pop up again at or close to the original site, e.g., herpes caught on your lip won't reappear below your chin. Herpes simplex is common; 50 percent of Americans test positive for the virus by puberty and 80 percent test positive by age 50.

Symptoms

If you've been in contact with the virus, symptoms usually appear within two to seven days (not everyone will catch it). With the initial infection, some people get flulike symptoms—for example, headache, backache, or a fever. Often there's tingling or itching of the skin followed by clusters of small, painful, fluid-filled blisters. With genital herpes, sores can be on the vagina, cervix, anus, penis, or other genital area, and there can be a burning sensation when you pee. The first episode may last two to four weeks, during which time the sores will scab over and then heal up. If you get a recurrence, these usually heal more quickly, within a few days, and rarely involve the flulike symptoms. A person is most infectious when they have sores, although four out of five sufferers get such mild symptoms they don't realize they have herpes. Mild symptoms can be a small cut, itchy patch of skin, or a pimple. Some people have the virus but may never get symptoms; others might not get their first attack until years after catching the virus. It's important to remember that the virus can be spread even if a person has no symptoms.

Tests and Treatment

Tests are done when the sores are present. Although there's no cure for herpes simplex (that goes for both facial and genital sores), an anti-viral drug, Acyclovir, can reduce the length and severity of attacks. Many people only get one or two attacks of genital herpes, but for some, it can return regularly, particularly when they're under stress or during their period. The virus can't be removed from your body. If you think you or your partner might have herpes, however mildly, it's important to get it diagnosed so that you can avoid sexual contact while there are sores.

Protecting Against Genital Herpes

Condoms can protect against herpes, but it depends where the blisters are. For example, if a boy has blisters on his penis, a condom will protect the girl as long as all his blisters are covered. But if a girl has blisters in her vagina, her partner might not be protected by a condom as her secretions, which may contain the herpes virus, can leak out over his body. Whoever diagnoses you will talk to you about how to prevent passing herpes on during sex. For more information, call the National U.S. Herpes Hotline (a long-distance call) at 1-919-361-8488 or visit the American Social Health Association Web site at http://www.ashastd.org.

Genital Warts

These are caused by a virus (human papilloma virus, or HPV). There are about a hundred different kinds of HPV, causing warts on the hands, feet, and genitals. Genital warts are common and are passed on during sex or by skin-to-skin contact. Only rarely can warts on fingers produce warts in the genital area, as they're different strains of the virus.

Symptoms

A person may have the wart virus in their body without any visible warts yet, but they can still pass the disease on. Or they may have tiny warts that aren't obvious, or ones in places you can't see easily. Girls can have warts in or around the vagina, vaginal lips, and cervix (womb entrance). Boys can have them on or inside their penis or around their testicles, but it's rare to get them around the mouth from oral sex. Both sexes can have warts on or inside their anus.

It can take from two weeks to a year or more for warts to appear after contact with the virus. Warts are usually painless and range from so tiny you don't notice them to flat, smooth bumps or large, pink, cauliflower-like lumps, on their own or in groups.

Tests and Treatment

The doctor can usually spot them, or they may wipe a weak vinegar solution over the area, which makes the warts turn white so they can be seen. To get rid of genital warts, the usual method is painting them with a chemical. They can also be frozen, heated, or removed by surgery or laser. Antibiotics aren't used, and ordinary wart treatments you can buy from pharmacies won't work.

It can take time to get rid of warts. Some people only get one episode, but others find they come back. There's no treatment to rid your body of the wart virus completely, but the longer you go without a reoccurrence, the less likely it is that they'll return.

Untreated warts sometimes go away on their own. However, if not treated they may get bigger or you may get more, and you can pass them on.

Protecting Against Genital Warts

Although condoms are good protection against most STDs, it's not clear how far they protect against genital warts. The best advice is to avoid sexual contact until visible warts have been treated, and seek help if you think you may have caught the virus.

Note: Genital Warts and Cervical Cancer

Some types of genital wart virus have been linked to changes in cervical (neck of the womb) cells, which could, in time, lead to cervical cancer. If caught early, these changes are easily treatable. All women over twenty-one should have a cervical smear test, called a Pap, every year, but if you've had genital warts, your doctor might suggest you have one earlier. Pap tests pinpoint any changes before they turn cancerous.

Gonorrhea

Gonorrhea (also known as the clap, drip, or sting) is caused by bacteria and is similar to chlamydia but less common. It's passed on by sex, including oral sex. This disease can cause serious long-term health complications if not treated.

Symptoms

Gonorrhea causes no symptoms in 10 percent of males and 50 percent of females. If you do get symptoms, they can come one to fourteen days after infection, or sometimes not until months later.

Girls: vaginal discharge that can be thin or watery and yellow or green in color; pain when peeing; lower abdominal pain.

Boys: white, yellow, or green discharge from the penis; pain when peeing; sore testicles.

Tests and Treatment
The doctor or nurse will take swabs from infected areas and possibly a urine sample. Gonorrhea is cured by antibiotics.

Protecting Against Gonorrhea
Use condoms whenever you have sex, including oral sex. Latex squares should be used for oral sex on a girl.

Hepatitis B

Hepatitis B is caused by the hepatitis B virus. It's more infectious than HIV and can be transmitted via sexual intercourse or contact with blood or blood-stained saliva and urine. It's not that common, but it isn't rare.

Symptoms
Some people get flulike symptoms and jaundice, in which the whites of their eyes and their skin turn yellow. Many get no symptoms.

Tests and Treatment
A blood test will show whether you have hepatitis B. You may be treated with a series of four shots of interferon, or by long-term treatment with pills such as lamivudine and adefovir dipivoxil. The best treatment is prevention. A vaccine is available from pediatricians and doctors and can be given anytime from infancy through adulthood.

Protecting Against Hepatitis B

Use condoms whenever you have sex, including oral sex. Latex squares should be used for oral sex on a girl. As hepatitis B is so infectious, you can catch it from kissing or sharing drinks or toothbrushes.

HIV and AIDS

AIDS stands for acquired immune deficiency syndrome, a collection of illnesses that occur because the body's immune (disease-fighting) system has been damaged by the human immunodeficiency virus (HIV). In the United States 930,000 cases of HIV have been reported and about 40,000 new cases are reported each year. Teens have the fastest increasing rates of HIV in the United States today. HIV is mostly passed on through sex without a condom. Bodily fluids containing enough HIV virus to infect someone are blood (including menstrual blood), vaginal fluids, semen, and breast milk. Saliva, sweat, and urine don't contain enough virus to infect someone, nor can coughs and sneezes pass it on. Drug users who share needles can pass on the virus, and a pregnant mother with HIV can transmit it to her baby before birth or afterward via her breast milk.

In the past in the United States, HIV was mainly transmitted between men who have sex with men. Recently though, the number of heterosexuals (people who sleep with the opposite sex) getting HIV has been catching up to cases acquired through sex between men, probably because many gay men have taken the safer-sex message seriously and are much more likely to use condoms than in the past.

Symptoms

When a person first gets infected with HIV, they may get a high temperature, swollen glands, and night sweats. After that, there's usually a long period—up to ten years or more—where there are no symptoms. But eventually, as the body's immune system gets weaker from fighting the HIV virus, the person gets an infection, such as pneumonia, that they can't shake off. That's when they may be tested and found to have HIV.

Tests and Treatment

The doctor or nurse will take a sample of blood to test. A person can't be tested for HIV until they've been infected for at least three months, as it takes that long for the body to produce evidence of HIV. The person can still pass HIV on to someone else during this three-month window, though.

There's no cure for HIV, although anti-HIV drugs can slow down the damage it does to the immune system. Better drugs mean people can live much longer with HIV, and feel much healthier, than ten years ago. Because of advances in treatment, people no longer get as sick, so the term *AIDS* isn't used as much anymore. Instead, doctors talk about "advanced HIV."

It used to be that someone with HIV would eventually develop AIDS and die, but because the combination drug therapies are relatively new, it's not yet clear what will happen to HIV sufferers in the long term. Their life expectancy is still likely to be reduced, depending on which strain of HIV they have and how they respond to drug therapy. HIV is still considered a fatal disease. Once a person has contracted HIV, they will always be infectious.

Protecting Against HIV

Use condoms whenever you have sex. Although there's only a small risk of getting HIV though oral sex, to be safe it's best to use a condom for oral sex on a boy and latex squares for oral sex on a girl.

Non-Specific Genital Infections (NSGIs)

This is a large group of infections that includes vaginitis (vaginal inflammation), urethritis (inflammation of the urethra, the tube you pee through) and proctitis (inflammation of the rectum). Not all of them are passed on by sexual contact.

Symptoms

There may not be any, but symptoms may include unusual discharge from the vagina in girls or from the anus or urethra (pee hole) in both sexes; sore or swollen genitals; pain or burning when peeing.

Tests and Treatment

Generally, the doctor or nurse will take a swab from the infected area. Treatment is usually with antibiotics.

Protecting Against NSGIs

Use condoms whenever you have sex, including oral sex. Latex squares should be used for oral sex on a girl.

Pubic Lice (Crabs)

These tiny insects live in coarse body hair, such as pubic hair. They don't live in head hair, but can also be found in chest, leg,

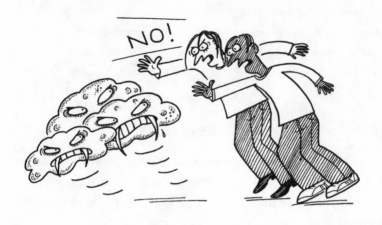

SAY "NO!" TO STDs!

underarm, eyelash, and beard hair. They don't fly or jump, but crawl onto other people. Pubic lice live on human blood but can survive for twenty-four hours off the body, which means that as well as being passed on through intimate contact, you can get them from clothes, towels, and bedding.

Symptoms

You may have no symptoms, or you might get itching; black, powdery lice droppings in your underwear; tiny brown eggs clinging to the hairs in the affected area; inflammation caused by scratching. The lice themselves are an eighth of an inch long, yellowy-gray, and look like tiny crabs. They can be hard to spot, as they keep still in the light.

Tests and Treatment

The doctor or nurse may take a magnifying glass to look for lice and eggs. Treatment is a special lotion, cream, or shampoo, and you don't need to shave the hair off. The treatment nearly always works. Pubic lice won't go away on their own.

Protecting Against Pubic Lice
Condoms don't protect against pubic lice. If you think you or your partner might have them, you should both have a checkup. Don't share clothes, bedding, or towels with anyone or have any sexual contact with your partner until you've both gotten the all clear.

Scabies

Scabies is caused by minute (a fraction of an inch long) mites that burrow into the skin and lay eggs. They're easy to pass on through sex or close bodily contact. Scabies mites can be around the genitals, between the fingers, on the feet, under the arms, around the buttocks, and on a girl's breasts. The mites can survive for seventy-two hours away from the body, so you can catch scabies from clothes, towels, and bedding.

Symptoms
You may not notice any symptoms, or you might get intense itching in the affected area that often gets worse at night or after a hot bath or shower. Scratching commonly causes cuts, and there may be an itchy rash or small spots. The mites are too small to see.

Tests and Treatment
The doctor or nurse can often tell by looking at the affected area, or they may take a flake of skin from a spot to check under a microscope for mites. Treatment is with a special lotion or cream. Scabies won't go away on its own.

Protecting Against Scabies

Condoms don't protect against scabies. If you think you or your partner might have it, you should both have a checkup. Don't have any sexual contact or share clothes, etc., until you've both gotten the all clear.

Syphilis

Syphilis (the pox) is caused by bacteria. Although syphilis isn't common, it's easy to pass on because symptoms can be so mild you may not notice them. It's passed on during sex and by skin-to-skin contact with someone who has syphilis sores or rashes. If not treated, syphilis can cause very serious damage to the heart, brain, lungs, eyes, and other organs and can be fatal.

Symptoms

Three to four weeks after coming into contact with the disease, you might get sores around your genital area or anus, which take several weeks to heal. If untreated, this is followed by a rash all over the body or in patches, flu-like symptoms, and tiredness. Symptoms can then vanish, but the disease is still there and you remain infectious.

Tests and Treatment

Tests for syphilis involve a blood sample and sometimes a urine sample and swabs taken from any sores. Treatment is by antibiotics and is very effective.

Protecting Against Syphilis

Use condoms whenever you have sex, including oral sex. Latex squares should be used for oral sex on a girl.

Trichomonas Vaginalis (TV)

Trichomonas is an infection cased by a tiny parasite, which is passed on via sex. Then it lives in the vagina and urethra (tube leading from your pee hole to your bladder) in women and in the urethra of men. Trichomonas isn't that serious, but it's often diagnosed alongside gonorrhea.

Symptoms

Up to half of all infected people don't have symptoms. However, up to twenty-one days after infection you could get a vaginal discharge that's thin and frothy with a musty or fishy smell; a sore, itchy vagina; a sore lower abdomen; and pain when peeing or having sex. Boys may get a thin, white discharge from their penis and pain when peeing.

Tests and Treatment

The doctor or nurse will take a swab from affected areas and may ask for a urine sample. Treatment is with antibiotics. These react with alcohol to make you feel really ill, so you cannot drink any alcohol during treatment. TV won't go away on its own.

Protecting Against TV

Use condoms every time you have sex.

WOMEN'S HEALTH

Bacterial Vaginosis (BV)

Also known as non-specific vaginitis, BV is cased by bacteria and is fairly common. BV occurs when the chemical balance of a woman's vagina alters—doctors aren't sure why—but it can also be passed to a woman during sex. Men can pass it on but tend not to get it themselves.

Symptoms

Often there are no symptoms, but if you get any, they'll involve changes in your vaginal discharge. It might get heavier or thinner, and/or become frothy, yellow, white, or greenish, and smell fishy, particularly after sex.

Tests and Treatment

The doctor or nurse will take a swab from your vagina and possibly a urine sample. BV is treated with antibiotics, or you may be given a cream to use in your vagina. Avoid alcohol if you're being treated with antibiotics, as those for BV react with alcohol to make you feel really ill. BV can go away without treatment, but if you get symptoms, it's best to get tested to be on the safe side, as you could have some other disease. It's quite common to get BV again.

Preventing BV

So you don't disturb the chemical balance of your vagina, avoid scented soaps, bubble baths, and vaginal deodorants and use milder soaps. Smokers are more likely to get BV because smoking disrupts the vagina's natural environment, leaving it more susceptible to BV bacteria. Always use condoms for sex.

Cystitis

This is very common, with at least half of all women and girls getting it at some point. Cystitis is an infection of the bladder, and although it's usually girls who are affected, boys can get it as well. Its main cause is bacteria that normally live in your bottom, which can easily be spread to your urethra (pee hole) and into your bladder. You can also get cystitis from the friction caused by lots of penetrative sex, known as "honeymoon cystitis." This infection is not truly a sexually transmitted disease.

Symptoms
Wanting to pee very often, which can feel as though you're bursting to go; burning or intense pain on peeing; unusual-smelling urine; cloudy urine; blood in the urine. Some women get a high temperature and/or abdominal pain.

Tests and Treatment
Often the doctor or nurse can diagnose cystitis from the symptoms, but they may ask for a specimen of urine to see exactly which bacteria are in your bladder. It's treated with antibiotics. Once you've had it you'll recognize the symptoms. Here are measures to take while you're waiting for the results of a cystitis test.

Cystitis Self-Help
* Drink lots of water (not tea, coffee, cola, etc.) to flush out the bladder and kidneys. For this reason don't delay going to the bathroom, even though peeing may be uncomfortable.

* Making the urine more alkaline soothes your bladder and helps to get rid of the bacteria. You can try one teaspoon of baking soda (find this in the baking section of supermarkets) in half a glass of water two or three times a day.
* Some girls find that drinking cranberry juice helps reduce the frequency of new infections and helps clear up active infections more quickly. Just make sure to drink a brand that contains at least 50 percent cranberry juice.

Make sure to see a doctor, as cystitis can spread to the kidneys and become more serious.

Preventing Cystitis

Drink at least 64 ounces of water a day. Always try to pee after sexual intercourse to flush any germs out of your bladder, and always wipe yourself from front to back when you go to the bathroom.

Pelvic Inflammatory Disease (PID)

PID is a bacterial infection usually caused by untreated chlamydia, gonorrhea, or other STDs spreading to the Fallopian tubes or other reproductive organs.

Symptoms

Anything unusual, but look out for bleeding between periods, fever, abdominal pain, and a tender cervix (womb neck).

Tests and Treatment

The doctor or nurse may know from your symptoms or take some blood to test. The underlying infection is treated with antibiotics. PID won't go away on its own. If not treated, women are at risk of constant abdominal pain and blocked Fallopian tubes, leading to infertility.

Protecting Against PID
Use condoms every time you have sex and seek help if you have any unusual symptoms, using those mentioned in the various sections of this chapter as a guide.

Yeast Infections (Thrush)
Also known as candida, a yeast infection is a condition that three out of four women will get at some point. It is caused by a yeast, *Candida albicans*, which lives harmlessly on your skin and in your mouth, stomach, and vagina. Sometimes, conditions change and the yeast multiplies and causes symptoms. For example, certain antibiotics can cause this infection, and it can crop up if you're under the weather. Although a yeast infection doesn't start off as a sexually transmitted disease, it can be passed on by sex.

Symptoms
Some people get no symptoms, but commonly there's a thick, white vaginal discharge with the consistency of cottage cheese and a yeasty smell like baking bread. You might also get itching, soreness, and redness around your vagina, vaginal lips, or anus; pain when you pee; pain during sex. Boys may get burning or itching under the foreskin or on the penis tip, along with red patches and a cottage-cheese-like discharge under the foreskin.

Tests and Treatment

The doctor or nurse will take a swab from affected areas and may ask for a urine sample. Yeast infections are treated with antifungal creams, pills, or vaginal suppositories (small tablets that you put up the vagina), sometimes in combination. Once you've had a yeast infection and know the symptoms, you can treat it yourself with cream and/or suppositories, such as Monistat, available from pharmacies. You can also smear plain yogurt containing bio-live cultures, or "friendly" bacteria (e.g., *lactobacillus acidophilus*)—also called "bio yogurt" (which you can find in some supermarkets, but it's easier to find in health food stores) on affected areas. This helps to restore the levels of "friendly" bacteria in the area (a panty liner will protect your underwear). Never use fruit yogurts, as the sugar in them feeds the yeast and will make the infection worse.

Preventing Yeast Infections

You might find certain things trigger this infection for you, so if you get one regularly, avoid wearing tight underwear and pants and fabrics made from synthetic fibers (yeast thrives in warm, moist conditions). Also avoid perfumed soaps, bubble baths, and vaginal sprays and deodorants, as these change your vagina's chemical balance.

Some girls report that being on the Pill gives them yeast infections. If this happens to you, keep taking your pills but see your doctor for treatment of the infection. Using pads rather than tampons during your period may also help, and always use condoms for sex. Wipe yourself from front to back after using the bathroom, and if you're prescribed antibiotics, tell the doctor that you get yeast infections. They may give you a yeast treatment at the same time.

Nutritionists recommend that all of us, whether prone to yeast infections or not, take a food supplement containing *lactobacillus acidophilus* (from health food stores), which restores the body's balance of healthy bacteria, during a course of antibiotics and for another week afterward.

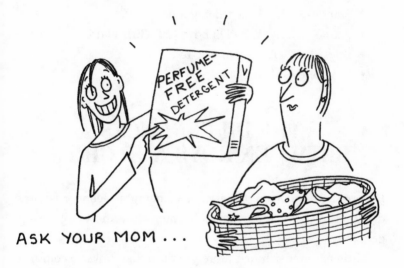

ASK YOUR MOM . . .

CHAPTER TWELVE
Boys and Sex

Next we look at what's going on for boys when they get together with girls. This chapter covers:

- The Differences Between Boys and Girls: Double Standards; It's Tough Being a Boy
- Name-Calling: Why Do Boys Call Girls Names?
- Boys' Top Ten Tales to Get You into Bed
- Boys and Girls on Dates

THE DIFFERENCES BETWEEN BOYS AND GIRLS

Experts agree that the experience of being a teenager is very different for boys and girls (as if you didn't know). Speaking generally . . .

Girls feel under much more pressure than boys to conform to a stereotype of body shape and attractiveness, whereas boys are "allowed" to come in all shapes and sizes. Short boys have a harder time of it, though, and practically every boy worries at some point that his penis is too small.

At first, girls are more likely to be confused and upset by the changes to their bodies, not the least because their boob size and looks in general are judged and commented upon. Boys, on the other hand, tend to grow in confidence as they get stronger and taller. Society in general and parents in particular panic about girls because they can get pregnant. This means that parents often mutter dark warnings to girls about the dangers of being alone with a boy, whereas teenage boys are given more freedom than girls and aren't advised to look out for themselves with the opposite sex.

Regarding friendships, girls tend to go for more intimate ones, where they share feelings and give each other support, whereas boys pal up according to activities they enjoy, like playing football. Boys tend not to discuss their feelings with each other, absorbing the message that it's sissified to do so. Often the first chance they have to explore how they feel with another person is when they get a girlfriend. Since girls are more experienced at feeling-talk, this is yet another reason why it might seem like an alien has been beamed down from Mars when you attempt to ask your boyfriend what's going on with him. If you get a series of grunts for an answer, don't assume he's being difficult. He's just not used to checking out his emotions.

While girls tend to talk about sex to each other at length and in a more serious, helpful way, boys are much more likely to boast, joke, and exaggerate what they're up to with girls as part of how they bond with each other. It makes boys feel grown-up and as though they know what they're talking about, plus it handily masks their fear of how uncertain they actually feel about the whole sex business.

Not only do girls mature earlier than boys physically, they also mature earlier emotionally. That means that a boy of fourteen might seem childish to a girl the same age, which is why girls often go for older boys. Luckily, boys catch up eventually!

Testosterone, the male hormone, contributes toward the sex drive in both males and females, but boys and men have much more testosterone than girls and women. (Incidentally, this doesn't mean that all boys and men have a higher sex drive than all girls and women—it varies between people.) When this hormone first starts swishing around in a boy's body, it results in frequent erections, often when they're least wanted, a raging sex drive, and sex on the brain much of the time. At first, boys satisfy these urges by masturbating, which they start earlier than girls, but soon enough their thoughts turn to real-life girls, which is where you come in. In their early teens, girls think about sex a lot too, but it's more likely to be in a romantic sense, and they're not so into the physical side at this stage.

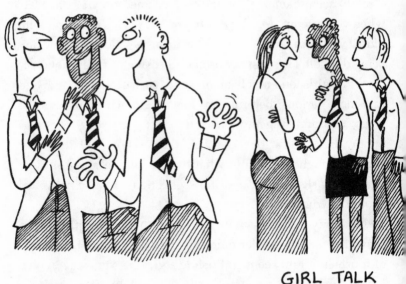

BOY TALK

GIRL TALK

Double Standards

The constant worry about whether they're thin enough, pretty enough, and filling their shirt in the right way means that teenage girls can lose some of the confidence they had as kids and find it hard to stand up for themselves against boys in sexual situations. It's easy to feel so grateful that a boy's paying you attention that you don't dare act like an equal in the relationship, even though you're far from doormat material with your friends. According to the National Campaign to Prevent Teen Pregnancy, 67 percent of teen girls receive the message that attracting boys and looking sexy is one of the most important things they can do.

Thanks to contraception, we don't have to risk making a baby every time we have sex, but the double standard is linked to a man's primitive drive to make sure he has descendants. Modern man (and woman!) has existed for about 100,000 years. Until paternity tests using DNA, which have only been around since the late 1980s, a man could never be certain he was a particular child's father, whereas you always knew who the mother was because she gave birth to it. This meant that the man who was fending for a mother and child could never be sure if he was putting his energies into bringing up his own or another man's child. So it would be in his best interest to impregnate lots of different women to make sure that, somewhere, a child of his was being brought up, while at the same time stopping the woman from sleeping around.

Although we don't think like this consciously, we're left with a vague idea that it's OK for boys to have as much sex as possible with lots of different girls but that for girls, sex should be with just one man, preferably the one they're going to marry and have kids with. Even though some things have changed, this still runs very deep in our culture, along with the notion that decent girls don't really want sex and have to be persuaded. I get lots of letters from girls who'd like to initiate sex with their boyfriend but worry that there must be something wrong with them for wanting sex when the boy doesn't (there isn't—it's perfectly OK to want sex if you're a girl).

It's Tough Being a Boy

Although girls come under pressure from media images of beauty, boys have their own issues, the main one being the pressure to "be a man" as soon as possible. For many boys, there seem to be two ways to go about this: find ultra-masculine role models to follow and forget about anything even remotely feminine. It's as if they can only work out how to be male by rejecting what's female. Any trace of "girlieness" in other boys is stamped out, which explains the popular pastime of calling each other "fag" or "gay" if they display anything other than macho behavior. Luckily, plenty of boys eventually understand that all of us have a mixture of both masculine and feminine traits, but the ones who don't realize this tend to grow into macho, homophobic men terrified of showing their tender feelings. They're not great to have a long-term relationship with.

Never underestimate the power a boy's friends may have over him. A new study from the Kaiser Family Foundation found that one out of every three teen boys reported feeling peer pressure to have sex—most often from male friends. So while boys are discovering love, sex, and emotions alongside girls, they're also trying to square up what they're feeling with what they need to do to win approval from their friends. This leads to the sorry situation in which a boy might be attentive and kind to you in private but ignore you or call you names when his friends are around.

NAME-CALLING

The worst thing for a boy is being teased about his sexual inexperience. Peer pressure means that boys who are way too immature to have a relationship wind up getting physical with a girl mainly to impress their friends. This is hard on the girl, because if the boy doesn't much care for her and is just with her because his friends think he should have a girlfriend, of course he's going to try to get as far as he can with her so he's got something to brag about. If you hitch up with one of these boys, you're damned if you do something sexual with him and damned if you don't, because either way you'll get called names, either to your face or behind your back. Common names include:

Frigid

This is an outdated term that used to appear in sexuality textbooks up until the 1970s, meaning a woman who didn't enjoy sex and couldn't have an orgasm. Nowadays, what a boy generally means when he calls you this is that you pushed him away when he tried to force his hand up your top. Boys who use "frigid" as an insult don't realize that the joke is actually on them for not having a clue about how to make a girl feel good emotionally or sexually.

Slut

A slut is supposed to be a girl who'll sleep with anyone and everyone. In reality, you can find yourself called this if you do anything (or nothing) sexual with certain boys and they then become angry with you for some reason. Calling you this is meant to make you feel so degraded that you're ashamed to show your face.

Skank

Skanks, according to some boys, are girls who aren't that attractive but who go around half-dressed and flirt like crazy in an attempt to attract boys. *Skank* is also used in the same way as *slut*, to mean a girl who sleeps around.

Dyke

Boys sometimes accuse a girl of being a lesbian, but use a more vicious and negative word, *dyke*, if the girl hasn't shown any interest in dating or sleeping with them.

Nympho

Short for *nymphomaniac*, sex researchers used to apply this term to women with a very high sex drive. This was in the bad old days when women weren't supposed to be interested in sex and were considered abnormal if they were as anxious to have sex as a man. So if a boy calls a girl a nympho, he generally means she was up for sex as much as he was, but that must mean there's something wrong with her. Needless to say, he's a sexist twerp. In reality, someone of either sex who beds lots of different partners is often doing it not because they adore sex but to fulfill some other emotional need, for example, to "prove" that they're attractive.

Why Do Boys Call Girls Names?

All name-calling says more about the person who's letting the insults fly than the person they're insulting. That said, it's very hurtful if someone's spreading cruel stories about you, and it's not always easy to rise above it. But whatever you have or haven't done, worrying about what other people think won't help. Sexual names like those just discussed are an attempt to control you and shame you into behaving in a certain way. Girls have been known to use them against other girls for this reason too.

The aim of all teasing and bullying is to get a rise out of the victim, so don't give name-callers the pleasure of seeing you lose your cool. Hold your head up high, let the gossips chatter, and stick with the people whose opinion really counts—the friends who love and support you. Soon your story will be yesterday's news and some other poor soul will be under the spotlight.

BOYS' TOP TEN TALES TO GET YOU INTO BED

Before I continue, remember: only you know whether or not you're ready for sex. Don't let anyone push you around.

One of the main issues between the sexes is that boys can be more detached about sex than girls. For example, boys are more likely to say they had sex the first time to see what it was all about, while girls more often claim it was because they were in love. For both sexes, sleeping with someone is far more satisfying if you like, even love, the person as well as trusting and getting along well with them, but even if a boy is truly smitten with you, curiosity, the idea that "sex is what boys do," and because they have frequent erections during puberty mean that often he's pushing for sex sooner than the girl. Let's face it, the question "Why don't we wait until we know each other better before we have sex?" isn't one you'd expect to come from the lips of your average teenage boy. Once the goal is in sight, some boys will try anything to get some action, including lying to you if it suits them. Here are ten of the most common lines they try, generally in a whiny voice, to persuade you to have sex:

1. You would if you really loved me.

This is particularly cruel, as it only works if you do love the boy. If you're told this, you're likely to feel guilty and like a heartless monster who's making her poor boyfriend suffer. As a zillion one-night stands the world over have shown, having sex with someone proves nothing, least of all that you love the person. You do that by showing them respect, care, and consideration and by not trying to blackmail them into sleeping with you when they're not ready. In other words, a boy who truly cares for you is content to go at a pace you're comfortable with. And anyway, you're in a relationship that will hopefully last a long time, so what's the rush?

2. I'm so turned on that it'll do me permanent damage if I don't come.

This old chestnut gets brought out when you've been getting up close and personal and he's got an erection as big as the Eiffel Tower. Some guys genuinely believe it'll do them harm if they don't ejaculate (the ache they get in their testicles is sometimes called "blue balls"). The fact is, yes, it's uncomfortable, but if a boy doesn't come, his penis will soon shrink back to normal and the feeling in his testicles will subside. Make it clear you have no time for blackmail such as, "But it's because of you, so it's only fair that you should help me out." It's not at all harmful, so don't feel under any obligation.

3. I'll dump you if you don't sleep with me.

Most boys don't put it as bluntly as this. Instead, they may mutter about how their last girlfriend slept with them on the second date, etc., but you both know what they're saying. Sadly, this is very common, but the thing to remember is that any boy who says or implies this is interested in sex for its own sake, not you. If he genuinely wanted to be with you, he wouldn't dare threaten you because he'd be too scared that you'd dump him for being a sexist, selfish user. And you'd be right to do so.

4. If you won't do it, I know someone else who will.

This is a delightful variation on "I'll dump you if you don't," which, again, a boy probably wouldn't put so bluntly. Instead, after he's tried and failed to shove his hand down your pants for the billionth time, you might, for example, spot him flirting with some other girl in the hopes that a touch of jealousy will make you do whatever he asks so you can hang on to him. Again, this boy's looking for someone to practice his sex moves on, and he doesn't care whether it's you or what's-her-name from up the road. Let him go. A boy who shows you this little respect isn't worth your time.

5. We're the only couple in our class who haven't had sex.

Whether you are or not, so what? You're all individuals, not a bunch of sheep, and you choose when to have sex on the basis of how you feel inside, not because of what everyone else is doing. They're probably all exaggerating anyway. Try pointing out sweetly how sad it is that your boyfriend is so lacking in confidence that he has to let his friends make his decisions for him.

6. Having sex will strengthen our relationship.

Another guilt trip to make you feel as though you're holding back from making a commitment to the relationship. But if you don't feel ready for sex, it's likely to be a miserable event that you'll regret, and you'll resent the boy for forcing you into it. Does that sound like a recipe for a stronger relationship to you? It's true that sex can deepen a relationship when you're both ready to take that step, but it can't save a relationship that's not working, nor will it make a boy fall in love with you if he doesn't already feel that way.

7. Let's just lie down together.

This golden oldie is responsible for many a girl with good intentions finding herself feeling pressured into having sex. Yes, it's lovely to cuddle up on the sofa or bed with a boy you like, and some boys might genuinely want to lie next to you and go no further. But often, a boy who tries this one is banking on you getting so turned on that he can sneak a hand in here and remove an item of clothing there, eventually persuading you to go all the way. If you know in your own mind how far you're prepared to go and you trust that your boy will stop when you tell him to, you could lie down with him. But given that so many first-time sex encounters happen because people got carried away and, as a result, didn't use any protection against pregnancy and STDs, it might be sensible to say, "No thanks!" in answer to this thoughtful suggestion.

8. I won't tell anyone.

It's a bad sign if a guy says this because it suggests he has an audience in mind waiting to hear the outcome of your encounter. Otherwise, why should the idea of telling someone even cross his mind, given that sex between two people is their business and no one else's? It also suggests there's something shameful about you doing it together, which is a bit worrying. If you have any reason to suspect that this boy plans to brag about what happens between you, you'd be wise to go no further.

9. Of course I love and respect you.

It's great to hear this from a boy who means it, but unfortunately there are guys who'll reel off this line simply to manipulate you into sleeping with them. Plenty of men and women approach sex from different points of view, with men being more interested in the physical stuff and women wanting emotional involvement first. So to speed things up, some boys might say they love you and tell you what you want to hear, then do a disappearing act. If you've only seen a boy a handful of times or if he treats you in an offhand manner and/or is unreliable, then it's not true that he loves and respects you, whatever he says, so tell him where to go.

10. You must be frigid if you don't.

This is a nasty, threatening thing to say, and any boy who comes out with this is to be avoided. No boy who cared for you even a tiny bit would dream of saying such a thing, and you'll regret it instantly if you sleep with someone who could treat you with such coldness and contempt. Sex is supposed to be about sharing a warm and loving experience, so don't waste your time on any boy who tries to make you feel there's something wrong with you and calls you names.

BOYS AND GIRLS ON DATES

After reading this chapter, you might be left thinking, "What's the point of even trying to get together with a boy when the picture's so bleak?" But don't despair. All the preceding are generalizations, and there will be plenty of boys (and girls) who don't fit these descriptions. Everyone's different, and all of us change throughout our lives as a result of our experiences. It's not helpful to try to slot yourself or others into a particular pigeonhole and then feel trapped by what you believe. Whether you're a boy or a girl, doing something just to look good in front of your friends is never going to make you happy. It's important to be true to yourself and make your own decisions.

For all their bravado and acting the Cool Dude, boys are as worried as girls are that they'll feel stupid and be ridiculed for not knowing what to say on a date or how to please their partner in bed. The way to a satisfying relationship has nothing to do with using the right lines or sexual techniques, and everything to do with communication. Learning how to tell each other how you feel and ask for what you want are what counts, and that's what you and your boyfriend will discover together that will make things special between you, including the sex if you choose to go ahead. We'll look at how to talk to him about sex in the next chapter.

CHAPTER THIRTEEN
Let's Talk About Sex

You want help and information, you want to check intimate stuff out with your friends, and you want to negotiate what to do and when with your boyfriend—but it can be hard to find the words.

Chapter 13 is all about how to talk about sex and relationships with the people that matter: your parents, friends, boyfriends, and those scary but mighty useful men and women in white coats, the health professionals. In turn, this chapter covers:

- Parents: Talking to Parents
- Friends: Peer Pressure; Talking to Friends
- Boyfriends: Talking to Your Boyfriend; Saying No
- Doctors and Other Health Professionals: There to Help; Confidentiality; Consenting to Contraception; Who to See for Contraception and Sexual-Health Advice; Visiting a Clinic; Calling Help Lines

PARENTS

You may think your parents are so out of touch with what it's like to be a teenager that there's no point trying to talk to them about sex, especially since it's so embarrassing. Your friends know where you're coming from, so why not just run things you're not sure of past them, rather than risk an argument?

Believe it or not, your mom and dad were teenagers once,

and they've probably been there and done that in situations similar to the ones you're worrying about. Not only can they be a source of reliable information about relationships and sex, but they can also offer support and advice. And if, heaven forbid, you do wind up with some major sex-related problem that you need adult help with, it'll be simpler to approach them if the channels of communication are already open on the subject, even if it's only a crack.

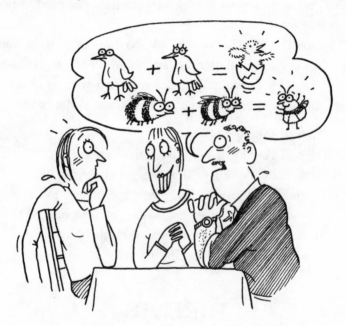

Talking to Parents

Apart from locking you in your room and throwing away the key, your mom and dad can't stop you from having sex if you're determined to do it. Since they're the grown-ups, it would be great if they could approach you in an open-minded way to discuss this tricky area, but plenty of parents keep quiet—not because they don't care, but because they think that you'll bring the subject up when you're ready. If they do begin a birds-and-bees-type discussion, resist the temptation to bury your face in a cushion and give them some help instead—it's your turn to be open-minded.

But it might have to be you who gets the ball rolling. Remember, your parents are just as uncomfortable about discussing sex with you as you are talking to them about it. For a start, parents panic that talking about sex is going to make you want to rush out and do it. (You can tell them that the opposite is true—kids who can discuss sex openly with parents are more likely to wait.) Also, many of them had an unsatisfactory sex education themselves, so they may worry that they can't answer specific questions. So be patient with them, and if they shy away from direct questions like frightened horses, ask something more general. Often they're scared that you're after personal information that they may not want to reveal about what they did. Here are some ideas on starting a discussion:

- Wait until they're chilled, in a good mood, and not distracted by something else, e.g. throwing dinner together or watching their favorite TV show.
- After talking about their day or whatever, ask a general question such as, "What do you think about sex before marriage?" rather than, "Can I go on the Pill so I can sleep with Dean?"
- Or you could mention something you've heard in sex ed or seen on a TV program, or show them a magazine article or this book and ask for their opinion. It's hard for parents to imagine their kids doing sexual stuff, so

be tactful about what you're up to.

- Then *listen* to what they say. Don't start yelling or storm out of the room if you disagree. This is a chance to show them you're a mature individual who's prepared to calmly consider both sides of an argument.

- Think carefully about what they tell you. Even if they seem overprotective, they do know the risks, so don't dismiss everything they say. They'll be more likely to take notice of what you say if you consider their points seriously.

- If they get mad, stay calm and make it clear you're only asking. Tell them that you want to be as informed as you can and think they're a solid source of reliable information. Showing your respect for what they say will win you a lot of Brownie points.

- Don't grill them in the hopes of getting details of a previous sex, drugs, and rock 'n' roll lifestyle. Leave it up to them to volunteer personal info if they want to.

- If you think one parent will be more receptive, approach *that* parent on their own. Don't be surprised if he or she tells the other one what you've said, even if they're separated. They both care about you and are responsible for you until you're eighteen.

- Unfortunately, some parents, for whatever reason, are never going to talk about sex with you, and that's a shame. If this applies to you, there are plenty of other adults around who could help, such as a relative, friend's parent, teacher, school counselor, or doctor. Also, you'll find a list of agencies you can approach in the "Resources and Contacts" section of this book.

FRIENDS

Some of us are lucky to have close friends we can discuss anything with, however embarrassing. But I hear from loads of girls who have questions about sex and relationships who say they would never ask their friends because they're worried their friends will think they're stupid. It feels as if everyone but them has the answers.

This is hardly ever true. If there's something you don't know, you can bet most of the people you hang around with are also clueless but too ashamed to admit it and so pretend they know instead. There's often a know-it-all in every gang who's actually misinformed and will even make things up to look clever. They wind up perpetuating the sex myths that get everyone confused.

Peer Pressure

Although this is more common with boys, girls come under fire from their peers too and wind up doing sexual stuff with boys to keep up with their friends. It's hard to escape this because we all want to be liked and be part of a group, but if you're getting it on with boys just to impress your friends, you're not going to make a very good girlfriend *and* you'll probably find yourself regretting what you've done.

Talking to Friends

First, I would seriously question how much of a friend someone is if they sneer at you for admitting you're worried or want information. Similarly, so-called friends who put you down and leave you out of things are going to make you feel bad about yourself, which is pretty sad since a good friend is supposed to do the opposite.

But often the pressure not to share our feelings comes from inside us. Everyone has insecurities, whether it's about sexual stuff, their bodies, their grades, or whatever, so if you have decent, reliable friends, take the plunge and tell them what's on your mind. Often you'll find they have the same worries. Having said that, if you're lucky enough to have loyal, loving pals, you don't need to be told how to talk to them because you're already doing it. But if you can't trust the people you hang around with, perhaps it's time to seek out a new friend or two. No one's perfect, but ideally you want someone who:

- won't blab about your personal info. You want someone you can be completely open and relaxed with, rather than having to censor what you say for fear it'll get spread around;
- is kind and considerate, and includes you in plans;
- shares secrets with you (which, of course, you keep to yourself);
- listens to what you say, is interested in you as a person, and wants to spend time with you alone and not just as part of a group;
- doesn't gossip about others—someone who does will gossip about you when you're not around;
- contacts you to go out as much as you contact her. If you're always having to chase someone, the relationship's out of balance, which puts you at a disadvantage.

It takes time to find out who's a good friend and who isn't. Life is hard without allies, but it only takes one loyal friend to make a huge difference. It might seem like a good idea to hang with the coolest girls, but in fact that girl you see around who doesn't say much might be in need of a friend and might make a more trustworthy one in the long run. There's a saying, "There are no strangers—only friends we haven't met yet." Why not talk to someone new today?

BOYFRIENDS

All the practical info in the world about protecting against pregnancy and STDs and when and how to have stupendous sex are of no use whatsoever if you can't communicate with your partner on these issues. Ironically, many girls find that the very person they should be able to discuss the basics of sex with, their boyfriend, is the hardest to talk to of all.

I've been seeing Simon for six months, and we're thinking of having sex. He's touched me around the genitals a few times, but he's quite rough and I don't enjoy it. I don't know how to tell him this without hurting his feelings, so I let him do it anyway. He doesn't want to use condoms because he says sex won't feel as good for him, so he says I should go on the Pill or something. I don't know if I want to, though. What can I do?

Abbi, 16

Talking to Your Boyfriend

If you think one or both of you might be ready for sex, it's sensible to sit down and discuss this as frankly as you can. Sounds obvious, but if you don't make your feelings clear, your boyfriend won't know what they are. He can't read your mind, however much you'd like him to be able to.

First of all, you have to know what you want to say. Forewarned is forearmed, so read this book a couple of times to get any arguments and thoughts straight in your head. Then if he says, for example, "Everyone knows girls can't get pregnant if their period hasn't started, so we don't need to use condoms," you can say, "Oh yes they can," and tell him exactly why. You might want to refer back to chapter 9, "Are You Ready for Sex?," for more ideas.

Vital topics for discussion include the following:

- Are you over the legal age of consent? You'll likely be more relaxed about the whole deal if you know you're on the right side of the law.
- What are you going to do about contraception? Does your boyfriend know that even if you go on the Pill, condoms should be used as well to protect against STDs?
- Will you go to the doctor or clinic together to sort out contraception? You can be seen together for this if you wish.
- If either of you have had any sexual contact whatsoever with another person (for example, touching their genitals or having yours touched or having oral sex), it's wise to get yourselves tested for STDs at a clinic before you do anything sexual with each other. You can go together, although you'll be seen separately.

It can be difficult enough communicating with the opposite sex, and there's added pressure when it's about something as intimate as sex. Even for girls who consider themselves to be pretty confident, it can be hard to find the right words. Below are some of the reasons for this:

- The words that describe the sexual parts of the body —for example, *penis, vagina,* and *clitoris*—can sound so clinical that it seems odd to use them. Similarly, the proper and slang terms for sexual acts, such as *fellatio* (oral sex on a boy—often called a *blow job* or *sucking off*), *cunnilingus* (oral sex on a girl—often called *eating her out* or *going down on her*), sexual intercourse (*screw, bang,* etc.) can seem, well, just plain *crude* and might make you feel dirty. Couples often get around this by inventing their own sexual terms that they're both comfortable with.

- Many boys and girls still believe that the boy should lead sex, and the girl has to put up with whatever he wants to do. Girls often feel they have no right to ask for what they want sexually, and that doing so will lay them open to charges of being a "nympho" or "slut." But the trouble is, if you don't say what you do and don't want, you'll end up, at best, not enjoying what happens between you and, at worst, suffering discomfort or having unsafe sex, as described in Abbi's letter.

- Another worry for girls is that her boyfriend might be hurt or even angry if she refuses sex, suggests they use condoms, or asks for something other than what he's doing to her. Perhaps he might even leave her. In reality, no boy who wants you other than just for sex will lose it if you say no. And a boy might be relieved that his girlfriend's mentioned condoms because he didn't know how to bring up the subject. Plus it's a huge strain on a boy to feel he has to know everything about sex and how to do it when he's probably as much in the dark as the girl is.

If there's something you think your boyfriend will be dead set against and you're worried whether you'll be able to stand your ground, try role-playing the situation first with a good friend. She can play your boyfriend while you play yourself. This can be more helpful than chatting to her about it, because, in character, you're more likely to come up with new solutions and ways of expressing yourself that you can then transfer to the real conversation.

Pick a time to talk to your boyfriend when you're both relaxed and won't be interrupted. Don't wait until things are getting hot and heavy.

Start with the basics:

1. Do you both feel ready?
2. What will you do about contraception and testing for STDs?
3. What will happen if you change your mind at the last minute? This is quite common, and you need to feel confident that your partner will be understanding if you get "cold feet" just before you're about to have sex and will be willing to stop.

When talking about your concerns, your likes and dislikes, and what you do and don't feel comfortable with, try to be as open as you can—but put a positive spin on things. This may sound dishonest, but it's just another way of saying the same thing and it works wonders. For example, would you prefer to hear, "Your bad breath makes me feel sick when you kiss me," or, "It's so good to kiss you after you've brushed your teeth and taste all minty and yummy"?

Often girls and women believe that their own pleasure comes second to their partner's and that if sex is enjoyable for them, it's by happy accident. Couples of all ages find that the woman expects to be passive and do whatever she's asked to satisfy her man. Speaking out can make you feel guilty, as though you're asking too much. But you have a *right* to feel just as good as your partner in bed, and don't let anyone make you feel otherwise. Pretending that you like what he's doing when you don't means he'll keep at it, thinking he's pleasing you.

Listen to what your boyfriend says and think carefully about how he sees things. Even in a strong relationship where you feel relaxed in your boyfriend's company, it can be hard going to persist until you reach agreements that satisfy both of you. Try to explore what it might mean to develop your relationship into a sexual one, and which kinds of sexual experiences you both enjoy and feel comfortable with or might like to try in the future.

Don't feel you have to cover everything and answer all your questions in one sitting. This isn't about reaching a "yes" or "no" decision about a one-shot experience; your discussions will be ongoing as you find out more about how you operate as a couple. Make sure you're both aware that if your relationship does become sexual, this doesn't mean you have to have sexual contact or intercourse every time you meet from now on.

All this talk makes sex seem like a serious business, which

of course it is in many respects. But at the same time, it's good if you and your boyfriend are so relaxed together that you can laugh about it when things don't go as smoothly as you expect them to. The most important thing is the relationship, and if that's good, sex will be the icing on the cake.

Saying No

If your boyfriend's pushing for sex and you decide that you don't want it, remember that you can say no. It's possible to refuse—even at the last minute and certainly before things get too heavy—without spoiling your intimate encounter or causing the relationship to end. One thing's for sure: you should never have to go further than you feel happy with. Here are some ideas about what to say:

- *"I really like/love you, but I'm just not ready to have sex."* This is perfectly reasonable. Make it clear that you're not rejecting him. This is about you, and you don't feel comfortable going all the way right now.
- *"It's too soon. I don't want to rush into anything."* Some couples wait one, two, or even more years before they have sex for the first time. Anyway, if you're in a long-term relationship, what's the hurry? There'll be plenty of time for sex in the future.
- *"I'd like us to get to know each other better before we go*

any further." Sex is better for both parties if you know and trust each other, and that takes time. You can still have fun and be intimate without having full sex.

- *"I'm too scared to have sex."* Pregnancy, STDs, breaking the law if you're underage, regretting having sex, finding it painful—all these things can be pretty frightening, and there's nothing wrong with admitting it. If sex really worries you, going ahead could turn you off to it for a long time.

- *"We don't have any condoms/contraception and I'm not taking any chances."* You're being sensible here—it's far too risky to go ahead without contraception or protection against STDs, so stick to your guns.

- There's nothing wrong with just saying, *"No, I don't want to,"* plain and simple, particularly if the boy is being very insistent. Make sure your body language matches your words so he knows you're serious. Move away from him, look him in the eye, and speak firmly, repeating the same "no" phrase if necessary. If you're not used to being assertive, practice saying no in other situations, like if your friend wants you to go somewhere you don't like.

Remember, if you don't want sex, clamming up or running away won't help. It's best to be straight rather than leave your boyfriend worrying about whether he's done something wrong or you don't like him anymore. Don't imply that you might change your mind any day now to get him off your back, unless it's true, or you'll have the same tussle every time you meet.

Chapter 15 is all about actually having sex and covers the first time and afterward.

DOCTORS AND OTHER HEALTH PROFESSIONALS

Doctors, nurses, and other health workers are particularly good to talk to about sex, contraception, and the like because they really know their stuff. The two most common reasons teenagers give for not seeking their help are (1) that they'll be reprimanded, and (2) that the doctor or nurse might tell someone else, such as their parents, that they visited. We'll look at each reason in turn.

There to Help

The medical people involved in giving contraception and treating STDs are on your side. If they weren't, they wouldn't be working in the sexual-health field! Family doctors, on the other hand, only prescribe contraception as part of what they do, so it might not be a particular interest of theirs. But whomever you consult, it's highly unlikely that they'll be anything other than cool and professional, whatever your problem or worry. If a medical person does make you feel uncomfortable, don't see them again—go elsewhere. Health clinics, such as Planned Parenthood, are particularly welcoming and friendly and understand exactly what freaks teenagers out about visiting clinics, so if you're scared about getting help, they're your best bet. If you're thinking of changing your family doctor, see the section about doctors on page 208 in "Who to See for Contraception and Sexual-Health Advice."

Confidentiality

In the United States each state has its own laws about confidentiality for teen medical treatment and teens' rights to consent for their own medical treatment. For the most part, teens have and can give informed consent and can receive confidentiality for birth control, pregnancy testing, prenatal care and counseling, testing and treatment for STDs, testing and treatment for HIV and AIDS, and sometimes abortion. You should check with your health-care provider before you begin treatment to clarify their policies on these issues.

Consenting to Contraception

* Teens can consent (agree) to their own treatment for contraception, if the doctor, nurse, or other health professional believes they're mature enough to understand the consequences of their decision. In practice, medical professionals generally feel that if you're sensible enough to ask for contraception, then you're mature enough to be given it. However, the medical person will probably try to persuade you to tell your parents, as this would be in your best interests, but they can't force you to.

* You don't usually need your parent's permission to get contraception, but it can be very stressful trying to hide the fact that you're having sex from them. Girls have been known to put their contraceptive pills in jars to disguise them, and then get all mixed up about which pill to take without the packet to guide them. It's better to be honest if you can. Your parents might not be as annoyed as you think and may even have helpful advice.

Who to See for Contraception and Sexual-Health Advice

Most doctors provide contraception and, if you can, it's a good idea to see your family doctor. They've known you a long time and have your medical history on file, which is important when it comes to working out whether certain types of contraception, such as the Pill, will suit you. They can also help if you think you might have an STD.

If you're too embarrassed to face your family doctor you have two choices: you can ask your parents to make an appointment with a gynecologist, or you can find a local health center. Contact Planned Parenthood at 1-800-230-PLAN for an appointment with the Planned Parenthood clinic nearest you. It is Planned Parenthood's policy to protect client confidentiality to the extent the law allows. Each state has its own laws about protecting teen confidentiality, so you'll need to check with your local health center to find out about local laws.

Visiting a Clinic

Some clinics you can just walk into and be seen, while at others you need an appointment, so call first to check. It's always a good idea to take a friend or partner with you for support. What happens varies depending on where you go, but most will ask for your name and address. This is for their records and won't be passed on to anyone. Then you'll meet a doctor, nurse, or other health adviser. If you'd prefer to see a male or female, say so.

- If you want **contraception**, the doctor or nurse will ask about your health and family history to make sure there's no medical reason why you can't use certain forms of contraception. Ask lots of questions to make sure you understand what you're being told. If you're under sixteen, they may suggest you tell your parents what you've decided. Confidentiality laws vary by state. You may want to check with the clinic when you make an appointment.

- Girls won't be given a vaginal examination unless they want an internal form of contraception such as a diaphragm, cap, or IUD. The staff will talk to you about protecting yourself against STDs, and then you'll be given your supplies of contraception, or a prescription to be filled at a pharmacy.

- If you want a checkup or treatment for **sexually transmitted diseases** (STDs), the doctor or nurse will want to hear about any symptoms. They'll also ask about your sex life, and it's important to be honest so they know how best to help you.

Then, depending on what the problem is, they'll examine you and take some samples. Your mouth, genitals, and skin may be looked at. Samples may be taken of urine, blood in some cases, or swabs from parts of the body that may be infected. A swab looks like a Q-tip and it's wiped over the area to pick up any discharge and skin cells. Samples are sent to a lab for checking, so you may have to wait for the results. All tests are optional. No one can make you have them.

You may get some treatment immediately, or the clinic will arrange for you to get the results of your test either by phone or in person and be treated later on. Ask lots of questions about how you might have gotten the STD, how you can protect yourself in the future, and the details of your tests and treatment.

Although laws vary from state to state, some STDs—like HIV, syphilis, and gonorrhea—often trigger mandatory notification procedures for sexual partners by health-care providers. Other times, it is up to each patient to notify previous sexual partners. Whether it is a legal issue or not, notifying your partners is always the right thing to do to protect their health and to prevent them from passing a disease on to other partners.

Calling Help Lines

There are help lines for every subject under the sun, from depression and drugs to heartache and herpes, and they can be a good starting point for assistance with something that's worrying you. Some give advice and information, while others have counselors who are trained to listen without judging you or telling you what to do. Avoid the premium-rate lines—they're just after your cash and will keep you hanging on for ages while you run up a huge phone bill. It's best to call only those you've gotten from a reliable source, such as books like this one, or magazines or Web sites you trust or that someone has recommended to you. (There's a list of helpful organizations at the back of this book.)

Help lines are great because you're in control, and if you don't like the way the conversation's going, you can hang up. Never give out personal information such as your name, address, and phone number unless it's a trusted source—for example, if you call Planned Parenthood for brochures. If anyone tries to pressure you into giving personal details, tell them you have to go and then hang up.

CHAPTER FOURTEEN

Test Your Sexpertise

QUIZ: ARE YOU A SEXPERT?

If you've read everything in the book so far, you're probably feeling a bit like a sex know-it-all. Dare you put yourself to the test to see what you've learned? Go on!

Have a look at the following statements and check whether you think they're true or false. Then turn the page to find out how you did.

1.	Condoms are available from family-planning clinics.	T	F
2.	Doctors can't tell anyone that you asked them for contraception.	T	F
3.	If you rinse your vagina with cola after sex you won't get pregnant.	T	F
4.	You can catch the HIV virus from kissing.	T	F
5.	You can get pregnant if you have sex during your period.	T	F
6.	You can't get pregnant the first time you have sex.	T	F
7.	There is a condom just for women.	T	F
8.	You're not a virgin if your hymen is broken.	T	F
9.	Oral sex is the term for talking dirty.	T	F
10.	If a guy has a hard-on and doesn't have sex or masturbate, it can be dangerous.	T	F

11. If you have unprotected sex, the emergency contraceptive pill only prevents pregnancy if it's taken the morning after.   T   F

12. Masturbating can damage or change the shape of your genitals.   T   F

13. The clitoris is located inside the vagina.   T   F

14. Condoms protect against STDs as well as pregnancy.   T   F

15. You can get pregnant from swallowing sperm.   T   F

How did you score? Give yourself one point for each correct answer.

1. **True.** 2. **True.** 3. **False:** There's nothing you can rinse your vagina out with that can stop you from getting pregnant, and anyway it can be harmful. Don't do it! 4. **False.** 5. **True.** Some girls ovulate (release an egg) during or just after their period. 6. **False:** you can get pregnant any time you have sex without contraception. 7. **True:** The female condom, is a small bag made of thin rubber that goes inside the vagina. 8. **False:** You're still a virgin until you have sex, whether your hymen is broken or not. 9. **False:** Oral sex is where you use your mouth on your partner's genitals. 10. **False:** It will do him no harm at all not to ejaculate (come). 11. **False:** The emergency contraceptive pill can be taken up to seventy-two hours (three days) after unprotected sex to prevent pregnancy. 12. **False.** 13. **False:** The clitoris is at the top of your inner vaginal lips. 14. **True.** 15. **False:** Sperm have to swim up your vagina for there to be a chance of pregnancy.

Look at the categories below to see what your score says about you.

5 AND UNDER: UNSURE ABOUT SEX

You know the basics of what goes where in sex, but that's about it. It's easy to make silly mistakes because you're not quite sure of the facts, so do yourself a favor and reread this book before you even think of going any further with a boy. Having the info at your fingertips will give you the confidence to join in when your friends are talking about sex and means you'll be able to stand your ground when the pressure's on, either from boys or your friends. Knowledge really is power!

6–10: SEX SAVVY

You're about average. You're clued in to many of the facts and will often be found explaining stuff to your friends. You understand a lot about your body and contraception, but your friends don't know that you sometimes get a bit muddled. Don't be tempted to ad lib to fill in the blanks, or everyone will get confused. There are holes in your sexual knowledge that you need to fill, so keep on reading and thinking things through, and you'll be a sexpert in no time!

11+: SUPER SEXPERT

Well done—you're truly knowledgeable about sex, bodies, and contraception. You know the facts and are happy to share them with your pals, and they know they can trust you as a reliable source of info. You may not have much experience yourself, but you've made it your business to get clued in on sex so you'll know what's what when the time comes. But don't let a good score go to your head: being clued in about sex doesn't automatically mean you're ready to plunge into steamy situations. Even the most sensible girls get it wrong sometimes, and this is one area where you can never know too much, so don't stop researching, asking questions, and mulling things over.

CHAPTER FIFTEEN
Having Sex

When you get to this point, ideally you and your partner will be at least sixteen and will have talked things over, weighed the pros and cons, and decided the time is right—you're going to lose your virginity. What can you expect?

This chapter covers:

- Before Sexual Intercourse: Kissing; Foreplay; Oral Sex
- Having Sexual Intercourse: Afterward: How Was It for You?; Will Sex Change Your Relationship?; You've Done It Once—Do You Have to Do It Again?; Orgasms
- Sex Myths Exposed

BEFORE SEXUAL INTERCOURSE

You'll have organized contraception and had tests for STDs if necessary. Now, rather than whispering, "I'm ready—go for it!" in your boyfriend's ear while you're cuddling, it's better to arrange when it's going to happen beforehand, so you can both be mentally prepared.

Foreplay is a vague term that baffles people, but it means intimate activities that get your bodies ready for sexual intercourse, i.e., the penis going into the vagina. At the very least, this will mean kissing, but it generally includes stimulating each other's genitals too.

Kissing

Lots of people aren't certain how to kiss, so we'll look at it here. Being literal about it, a kiss is where you press your lips against a person's skin or lips, and in French kissing, you move your tongue around in their mouth. You could say that making out is a bit of both. In reality, sloppiness and shoving your tongue down your partner's throat are major turnoffs. Instead, when a boy goes to kiss you, part your lips a little, then use your tongue lightly, as though you're tasting his lips and tongue. If you're mutually responsive, the kissing gets deeper as you both open your mouths wider. It might sound a bit nutty, but kissing works best when each partner responds to what the other's doing, like dancing together. As with all intimate contact, kissing's less about technique and more about your feelings for each other. The world's greatest kisser won't float your boat if you don't like him.

Foreplay

This is any activity that turns you on and gets you in the mood for sex. Its purpose is to make the boy's penis erect and the girl's vagina start to secrete the special liquid that acts as a lubricant to help the penis slide in. In reality, boys usually get an erection very quickly, but girls can take much longer to warm up. Foreplay can include stroking, handling, and kissing any part of the body that feels good. For girls, the center of their sexual universe is generally the clitoris, but it's so sensitive that it hurts to touch it directly until they're pretty turned on. For boys, it's stimulation of the penis.

Foreplay doesn't have to lead to actual sexual intercourse.

Often it's pleasurable enough in itself, and both partners can have an orgasm through having their genitals played with if they want to. Having said that, it's advisable always to have condoms handy if you're likely to get into a steamy situation. Even the most sensible of girls have ended up getting carried away without meaning to, and you don't want to wind up wishing you hadn't gone the whole way or, even worse, land yourself with an STD or unwanted pregnancy.

For instructions on how to put on a condom, flip back to chapter 10, "Contraception." The condom goes on as soon as the boy's penis is erect, before it goes anywhere near the girl's genital area. Lots of couples make putting on a condom part of foreplay.

Oral Sex

Using your mouth on your partner's genitals (oral sex) isn't something that everyone is comfortable with, but some couples enjoy it. Many girls worry that there's some special technique for performing oral sex (a blow job) on their boyfriends that they must master before they attempt it, but like all sexual activities, you'll learn what to do together, and in this case your boyfriend will guide you on what feels good.

Some girls are fearful of having oral sex performed on them because they're convinced that their genitals smell and that will put the boy off. In fact, many boys (and girls) like the scent of clean genitals. And the lips and tongue, being wet and soft but muscular enough to exert firm pressure, can often produce orgasms in girls who find it hard if not impossible to come from exploring fingers and straightforward intercourse.

HAVING SEXUAL INTERCOURSE

Before a couple can have sexual intercourse, the girl must be turned on enough, otherwise her vagina will be too dry to allow the penis to enter it. Sex really does start in the head, and the more nervous the girl becomes, the less likely it is that she'll become lubricated, which is why it's vital that she's content with and relaxed about what's going on. If the penis won't go in, couples can try kissing and cuddling for a while to see if the girl becomes more lubricated. It's sometimes better to try sex again another day rather than to forge ahead and cause the girl so much pain that she's repulsed by the whole situation.

For the first time, many couples go for the missionary position, where the girl is on her back with the boy kneeling between her legs. The penis won't float into the vagina of its own accord. Either the girl or the boy, or both, need(s) to guide it in with a hand. Gentle thrusts of the penis will help to open up the vagina, as it is a sensitive area that's not used to having anything as big as a penis in it. If the girl's hymen is still intact, she may feel a sharp pain as the penis pushes through it, but it certainly isn't agony and there won't be gushing of blood. Some girls bleed a small amount, which will soon stop. If you're worried about stains, put an old towel under you.

The boy then rhythmically pushes his penis in and out of the vagina, and the girl often meets his movements with her hips. Your first experience of sex is over when the boy has ejaculated (come). That's because he can't keep thrusting once this has happened, as his penis will go limp. It's unusual for a girl to have an orgasm the first time she has sexual intercourse, but if she wants one, she or her partner can help her have one afterward. When the sex is over, both partners tend to feel relaxed and cuddly and want to snuggle up together.

Afterward: How Was It for You?

You've probably been talking about, planning for, and panicking about losing your virginity for ages, but rather than fireworks going off and a hallelujah chorus serenading you from above, often the event itself is a bit of a letdown, particularly for the girl.

Some girls feel the physical effects of intercourse for several days afterward. It might be that the foreplay was rushed (or there wasn't enough of it) and you didn't produce much vaginal lubrication or you weren't relaxed enough. You can end up feeling sore or uncomfortable, and this can lead to worries that you've damaged yourself. As always, it's worth getting checked out by your doctor if you're particularly concerned.

For some people—and this is most common in boys—sex is a purely physical thing with very little emotional involvement. Once they've come, it's like a switch is thrown inside their head and they lose interest in their partner. One boy, Joe, admits that after he got badly hurt by a girl, he began to look at sex in that way:

Me and my friends find that so many girls nowadays are happy to have sex with you very quickly. It's like they spot a guy who dresses well and has some money, and they think you'll fall in love with them if they give you sex. No way. A lot of girls think you're their property and they can call you every day and find out what you're doing just because you've slept together. That turns me off even more. So I say to girls, don't judge a book by its cover. Don't think that good looks equal a decent guy.

Joe, 18

Or it could be you who can't face your partner afterward. A common reason is because you didn't know the guy too well and now feel so embarrassed by what happened between you that you want to avoid him. This is cruel if he likes you. A useful rule is to always treat others in the way that you'd want to be treated.

As Joe points out, sometimes boys and girls do approach sex wanting totally different things. But there's no shortcut to finding out whether you have the same outcome in mind—the key is to spend lots of time together and discuss your fears and fantasies.

Will Sex Change Your Relationship?

Ideally, you and your boyfriend, having shared such an intimate experience, will find your relationship getting deeper and stronger over time as your commitment to each other grows. It's true that having sex with someone you love deeply and who feels the same way about you can be a truly wonderful experience. At the other extreme, unfortunately, sex with the wrong person or at the wrong time can be one of the most painful things that can happen to you, so it's important to do all you can to ensure the circumstances were right for you.

Sex generates incredibly strong emotions and can leave you feeling vulnerable and mixed up. For example, you might suddenly feel emotionally dependent on your boyfriend in a way you didn't before. Having sexual intercourse is likely to change the way you see yourself, as the messages—both good and bad—that you've absorbed from parents, friends, the media, etc., about girls who have sex come back to you. Talking to your boyfriend and best friend about your changing feelings will help you come to terms with them.

It's important to never forget that whenever you have sex, there's always some chance of pregnancy, as no contraception is 100 percent foolproof. That's not to say that you should start arranging a mortgage and the wedding ceremony quite yet, but if you're planning to have sex regularly, you both need to be prepared to explore what you might do if you did get pregnant.

Sex isn't something that you get wrong or right, like a math problem. It takes practice to get the most out of sex, and after the first few times, you'll both become more confident as you find out how to please each other. Soon enough, you'll find you're enjoying sex more.

You've Done It Once—Do You Have to Do It Again?

Definitely not. It's your body, and you have every right to choose to say no next time the question of sex comes up. It could be that, this first time, you'd been drinking and weren't in full control of yourself. Perhaps you got carried away in the heat of the moment. Or perhaps you felt under pressure and said yes when, down deep, you meant no, but couldn't quite work out how to call a halt to the proceedings. Maybe you didn't enjoy the experience at all and feel like putting it off for a while. Whatever the reason, if you wish you hadn't gone all the way, you can't take it back, but you can decide not to have sex again for the time being. And the next time may or may not be with the same boy.

The trick is to be sure in your own mind what you want and don't want. That way you're less likely to be open to persuasion. It's perfectly reasonable to say something like, "It was great being so close to you, but I wasn't quite ready and I'd like to go back a few steps. It really wasn't anything you did—it's about how I feel." Your partner might not like it, or he might agree that the time wasn't right. If he's unhappy, reassure him that you can still enjoy kissing and cuddling and, if you feel comfortable with it, foreplay. If it's what you think, let him know that there'll be plenty of time for sex in the future—just not right now.

There's no reason why you should have sex every time you and your boyfriend meet. In the same way that not everyone is hungry at the same time, there will be occasions when one of you wants sex and the other doesn't. Learning how to deal with differences in desire are all part of negotiating a mature sexual relationship.

So what about with your next boyfriend? Some people think that, just because they've had sex with one person, they might as well hop into bed with everyone else they go out with. But it's not true. Every relationship is different, and you need to think through how you feel about each new person. In fact, it can feel like the first time all over again! Only *ever* have sex if you genuinely feel that the time, place, and person are right— and if you're prepared when it comes to contraception.

Orgasms

It's not true that the best sex is where both partners orgasm at the same time. While it's nice if it happens occasionally, in practice it's hard to pull off because boys and girls need different sexual stimulation to have an orgasm. With boys, movements up and down the length of the penis, provided by a hand or thrusting in the vagina, brings them to orgasm. But for a lot of girls, their clitoris has to be stimulated in the right way for them, and the movements of the penis during sexual intercourse hardly ever provide this. Only about one in three girls and women can have an orgasm through intercourse alone. If they like, the boy or girl can stroke her clitoris during intercourse, and that can result in an orgasm.

Forget the films and books that show women screaming and thrashing about like wild horses when they orgasm. Sure, some girls like to move about during orgasm, but others like to stay still. And some may shout, cry, or moan, while others are silent. It's your orgasm, and as you learn to let go, you'll find out what's natural for you. Some girls find that sexual stimulation straight after an orgasm will result in one or more further orgasms. This is called multiple orgasm.

SEX MYTHS EXPOSED

You look different once you've had sex and everyone can tell.
It's not true that you walk differently or have a special "Guess what I did last night?" look about you. The girl might feel a bit sore around her vagina for a few days, and her inner thigh muscles might ache for a day or two due to stretching her legs wide. The boy might find his arm and stomach muscles ache from the effort of holding himself up. None of this will be obvious to other people, though.

Lots of sex gives a girl a big, baggy vagina.
No, it doesn't. The vagina expands to hug any size of penis and, after sex, it simply goes back to its usual state, which is with the walls touching each other. Some women find that pushing a baby out through their vagina stretches it a bit, but luckily penises are a lot narrower than babies' heads, so this isn't

something you need worry about right now! There are vaginal exercises a woman can do after she's given birth, so this generally doesn't cause problems anyway.

The bigger a boy's penis, the easier it is to satisfy a girl in bed.

This is every boy's fear—that they won't be big enough to please a girl sexually. But how much a girl enjoys sex has very little to do with the size of a boy's penis, and everything to do with how it's used and how much attention he pays to ensuring she's getting pleasure from the other stuff he's doing. The vagina's nerve endings are concentrated at the entrance, so once the penis is in, the sensations are pretty similar whatever the size of the penis. And a truly enormous penis is actually a bit scary, as it can hurt when it goes in, although the vagina does expand to accommodate any size of penis.

Alcohol makes you want sex and relaxes you.

This is true in the sense that knocking the drinks back reduces your inhibitions and makes you less shy, so you might agree to do things you're less likely to do sober—like jump into bed with someone. But the problem is that even a few drinks stop you from thinking clearly, so you may well do things after a drink that you really wish you hadn't—like having unprotected sex or sex with a boy you don't like. Many a girl has lost her virginity while under the influence and lived to regret it, so don't let that happen to you. Lots of booze makes you sleepy, so you might find yourself feeling horny but too tired to have sex or an orgasm. Boys often can't get an erection at all if they've been drinking.

CHAPTER SIXTEEN
Sex—When You Don't Want It

It's a sad fact of life that there are people who don't respect others' boundaries and enjoy the feelings of power that come from sexually harassing, abusing, or assaulting others. This chapter looks at the main areas of unwanted sexual attention, what you can do to lessen your chances of being preyed upon, and what to do if you are targeted. It covers:

- Sexual Harassment: Flashers
- Sexual Abuse: What to Do if You're Being Abused; What if You Choose to Do Sexual Stuff with Someone Older Than You?
- Sexual Assault
- Rape: Date and Acquaintance Rape; Pressure from Boyfriends to Do Sexual Stuff; "Date-Rape" Drugs
- Sexual Assault and Alcohol
- What to Do if You've Been Sexually Assaulted or Raped
- Feelings After a Sexual Attack
- Helping a Friend Who's Been Attacked
- Staying Safe: Avoiding Drug Rape; Keeping Safe While You're Out; Safe Dates; Net Know-How

SEXUAL HARASSMENT

Some boys and men think it's funny to call you sexual names, proposition you, ask about your sex life, or put pornographic pictures on your desk at school or work to see your reaction. And while some girls and women join in with this, seeing it as part of the flirting and bantering that goes on between the sexes, others are deeply distressed by it. When it's extreme, it's a form of bullying that can be intimidating and humiliating and can lead to loss of confidence and even major depression.

If you've asked the person or people to stop and they persist, or if you feel too scared to confront them, you'll need to tell someone in authority who can help you. You don't have to put up with this, whatever anyone says. Challenging what's happening is *not* making a fuss about nothing.

- If this happens to you at school, tell a teacher you trust and your parents, or someone else in the family. Write a note if you can't face talking about it and give it to the person you've chosen to help you. Many schools have antibullying policies, but whether yours does or not, your school needs to know so it can step in and sort things out. To talk or get advice, visit Stop Bullying Now! at http://www.stopbullyingnow.hrsa.gov or call the National Youth Violence Prevention Resource Center at 1-866-SAFE-YOUTH.
- If it happens at an after-school job, sexual harassment is a form of sex discrimination and you have a legal right not to tolerate it. Report the harassment to your employer. If that doesn't work or the person who's

bothering you owns the company, you can take the matter to the U.S. Equal Employment Opportunity Commission at http://www.eeoc.gov.

Flashers

Unfortunately, lots of females experience a strange man flashing his penis at them at some point. While some girls and women laugh it off, many find it very upsetting, partly because of the fear of what the flasher might do next. But the stereotype of the sad old geezer in a dirty trench coat is wrong. Flashers tend to start in their teens and carry on throughout their life if not treated. And although a flasher is unlikely to touch you, experts have found that they do, over time, move onto more serious sex crimes if not caught and treated.

If a man flashes you, try not to react, as that's what they want—it means they can pretend to themselves that you secretly enjoyed it. Despite its jokey seaside postcard image, flashing is not trivial, so tell someone you trust and report it to the police. Exposing the genitals in this way is a crime, and if the man is caught, with luck he'll be prevented from flashing or harming others in the future.

SEXUAL ABUSE

Not unlike the flasher, the image we have of an abuser is some nasty-looking man lurking in the park offering kids candy. Not so. Someone you know, trust, or even love is far more likely to abuse you than a stranger. It could be a blood relative—dad, cousin, grandparent, uncle—a stepbrother or stepfather, or a schoolmate, teacher, babysitter, or neighbor. Some abusers are women. Anyone older, stronger, bigger, or with authority over you who does something sexual to you or in front of you is sexually abusing you if you haven't consented. This applies even if they're your age or a family member. And it includes talking dirty to you or getting you to look at porn. Taking kids out, buying them presents, and showing them porn is part of "grooming," or getting them ready to do as the abuser says.

Giving your consent—choosing whether to say yes or no to what's going on—is complicated in an abuse situation. If you're scared the abuser will hurt you or your family or won't listen even if you do say no, you might keep quiet or agree to the abuse out of fear.

Abusers believe what they're doing is OK and aren't interested in how you really feel. They're clever and know how to manipulate you into keeping quiet: for example, they may target lonely kids or get those they're abusing to hurt younger children so they'll feel guilty and keep everything secret. Commonly, they'll insist you really like the abuse and even gave them the come-on, saying that it's you who'll get into trouble if you tell or that telling will make family members ill or break up the family. Be aware that your body might respond to sexual touches even if you hate what's going on, which can make you feel very confused and guilty.

What to Do if You're Being Abused

Initially, adult abusers may seem kind and concerned, spending time building up a relationship with you before the abuse begins. Abusers make all manner of threats to stop you from telling, often insisting the abuse remain a secret between the two of you. But you have nothing to be ashamed of, and it's *never* your fault if you've been abused.

Whether it happens once or is ongoing, being abused can have serious long-term effects. Victims can find themselves suffering from depression, eating disorders, alcohol or drug addiction, and have trouble trusting people enough to develop close relationships. Sharing your feelings via counseling can be an important step in rebuilding your life after abuse.

However scared you are, you can get the abuse stopped, but you have to *tell someone*. It can be hard to ask for help and you may have mixed feelings, particularly if it's someone you love, but you don't deserve to be abused. What you do deserve is help and support, and there's lots of help out there.

- Tell an adult you trust, and if they don't take you seriously or don't do anything, tell someone else. Keep telling until someone helps you.
- If you can't face talking about it, write it down and then show it to the person you've chosen to ask for help. Or talk to a friend first and practice what you'll say. You could take your friend along while you tell.
- If none of the adults you ask are helpful, or if you'd prefer, you can call the police and say you want to talk to someone about child abuse. You can formally report what's happening or you can remain anonymous and just get advice. Depending on your age and the details of the abuse, they may suggest you let them step in and help, but they won't force you.
- If you just want to talk to someone about what might happen if the abuse is formally reported, or for general advice on stopping the abuse, information, and counseling, call Childhelp USA at 1-800-422-4453 or visit their Web site at http://www.childhelp.org.

It can take a long time, years in some cases, for a person to recognize that what happened to them was sexual abuse. Offenses that took place a long time ago may still be prosecuted depending upon the laws of the state where the crime occurred.

What if You Choose to Do Sexual Stuff with Someone Older Than You?

I've liked my math teacher for two years, and I'm really happy because he recently told me that he feels the same way about me. He says we can start going on dates soon, although we won't have sex until I'm at least sixteen. We're not breaking the law, are we? I don't want him to get into trouble. He's twenty-six.

Zuleka, 15

I get quite a few letters like Zuleka's, where a young girl likes an adult, such as a teacher, and assumes it's OK to do sexual things with him because she wants to, that is, she gives her *consent* (the legal term for agreeing to an activity). But in fact, teachers, youth leaders, the staff of children's homes, stepparents, probation officers, and other adults who are in positions of authority are dealt with very harshly by the courts if they indulge in *any* sexual activity with teens in their care. That means that even if you've reached eighteen, the person in authority is breaking the law. They're guilty of sexually inappropriate conduct, even if the young person consents, and the younger he or she is, the stiffer the adult's prison sentence will be. The grown-up is held responsible because they're expected to be able to control their own urges and not use their adult power to manipulate a younger person.

If an underaged teen agrees to sexual touching or penetrative sex with an adult (i.e., someone over eighteen) who isn't in a position of authority (for example, a twenty-year-old neighbor), the adult is still committing a crime. Any adult who has penetrative sex with a youngster under thirteen, even if the youngster agrees or the adult thought the youngster agreed, could be imprisoned for life.

SEXUAL ASSAULT

No one has the right to grope or touch you sexually without your permission, whether at school, work, or anywhere else. If you, or someone you know, has been a victim of sexual assault, confide in a trusted adult, contact The National Center for Victims of Crime at http://www.ncvc.org, or call 1-800-FYI-CALL.

Regarding serious offenses, see "What to Do if You've Been Sexually Assaulted or Raped," on pages 234–236.

RAPE

There are all kinds of myths about rape: that it's due to men's uncontrollable sex drive; that only young, sexy girls get raped (and they must have been asking for it anyway); and that most rapists are strangers lying in wait in dark alleyways. None of this is true.

- Men can easily control their sexual urges, and the vast majority do. Rape is about violence and power over another person, not about sex. Rapists actually admit this.

- Women, children, and men of all ages (including babies and the elderly), racial groups, and classes have been raped.
- What a girl or woman is doing or wearing makes no difference—no one deserves to be humiliated and forced to commit sexual acts against their will. Many rapes are carefully planned.
- For teens and college sudents, in over ninety out of a hundred cases of rape, the person knows their attacker. Around half of all rapes happen in the victim's or attacker's home.

Rape is defined as penetration by a penis of another person's mouth, anus, or vagina without their consent. Research suggests that less than half of all rapes are reported to the police, with date rape (see below) much less likely to be reported than rape by a stranger.

You might hear people say that because a girl or woman didn't struggle during the attack, it wasn't rape and she consented. This is untrue and is simply another way of shifting responsibility for the attack onto the woman. The fact is, many women are too terrified to struggle or make any noise during an assault. Following from this, not all rapes involve outright violence. Some boys or men take advantage of a girl or woman who is unable to speak up because she's drunk or on drugs.

Date and Acquaintance Rape

So-called date rape is carried out when the girl or woman chose to go on a date with the boy or man but was then raped. Attackers can include current or ex-boyfriends, boys met on the Internet, or pen pals—anyone you might go on a date with.

Acquaintance rape is where the attacker was known to the girl or woman but not a close friend, for example, her teacher, doctor, youth worker, or friend's boyfriend.

With date and acquaintance rape, the victim is often confused by what occurred and can't quite believe she was raped by someone she knew and, in many cases, trusted. It can take a while, sometimes months, for the truth about what happened to her to sink in. This kind of rape, rather than rape by strangers, is the most common form of rape. In fact, 67 percent of all sexual assaults in the United States were committed by someone known to the victim. Boys or men who carry out this kind of rape will usually say that the girl or woman consented.

Pressure from Boyfriends to Do Sexual Stuff

Not all circumstances where girls wind up doing sexual stuff they don't want to arise where there's an obvious power imbalance. It can be far more subtle than that. When we're going out with someone, ideally we'll only get intimate or have full sex because both partners want to at that time. But we don't live in an ideal world, and some girls find themselves in a situation where a boyfriend's desire for sexual gratification is so strong that it blinds him to the fact that she doesn't feel the same way. In particular, this might crop up if a couple has been intimate or had sexual intercourse before.

It might be tempting to make life easy and give in, but bear in mind that if you do, you'll be setting up the expectation that your boyfriend can have sex with you whenever he wants and your wishes will become less and less important to both of you. Never forget that it's your right to refuse if that's how you feel, and it's far better for your relationship and your self-esteem if you learn to stand up for yourself. For tips on how to do this, refer back to the section "Saying No" on page 204.

"Date-Rape" Drugs

Known as "date-rape" drugs but more properly called "drugs used in drug-assisted rape and sexual assault," these are substances that are dropped into your drink without your knowledge to make you so out of it that someone can rape or sexually assault you without you struggling. There are several date-rape drugs around, the best known being Rohypnol and GHB, but the street name for all date-rape drugs is "roofies." They're often tasteless and colorless and aren't just added to alcohol. Tea, coffee, cola, milk, and milkshakes can all be spiked.

To onlookers, the drugged person appears drunk, staggering and slurring their speech. While the rape or assault is taking place, a victim is dimly aware of what's going on but powerless to stop it, although as the drug gets deeper into their system, the memory of the event is lost for several hours, depending on the drug. Generally, these drugs disappear from the body within hours, with the precise time depending on the drug (for example, Rohypnol is absorbed within forty-eight hours, but others can take much less time), which means that by the time the memory of the rape or assault has returned, often there are no traces of the drug left in the person's body to use as evidence.

If you wake up in a strange place, or even at home (some victims are taken home and raped), with your underwear scattered around, sore genitals, or physical evidence of sex, but have no memory of anything happening, you may have been drugged and raped or assaulted. Follow the advice given in "What to Do if You've Been Sexually Assaulted or Raped" (see below). To press charges, go to the police as quickly as you can and ask them to take a blood and urine sample in the hopes of catching evidence of the drug before it's absorbed into your body. Remember, the police will treat you as a rape victim rather than try to prosecute you for drug taking.

SEXUAL ASSAULT AND ALCOHOL

Despite all the panic about date-rape drugs, experts are quick to point out that alcohol alone is a factor in many rapes and sexual assaults, with the attacker, victim, or both having been drinking. People who plan to take advantage have been known to ask the bartender to add a double shot of vodka, for example, when buying a girl a drink, and you probably wouldn't realize extra alcohol had been added.

We all need to be sensible around alcohol and not take unnecessary risks. According to Bureau of Justice statistics, in 2004, two in every five college campus rapes involved drugs or alcohol. Know your limits, alternate alcoholic drinks with soft drinks, and if you start to feel drunk, stop drinking and ask a close friend to get you home or call your parents. Better to get a lecture than be attacked.

But remember, even if you've been drinking or taking drugs and are attacked, it still isn't your fault.

WHAT TO DO IF YOU'VE BEEN SEXUALLY ASSAULTED OR RAPED

Being sexually assaulted or raped is extremely traumatic and the last thing you may feel like doing if you've suffered this is going to the police. You may even doubt what happened to you. It's your choice whether you report a rape or sexual assault, and if you go ahead, it has to be said that there's no guarantee the person who attacked you will be prosecuted. Police training has improved hugely in this area, and you can now expect to be taken seriously and treated with sensitivity at the police station.

- At the very least, you'll need medical attention. If there was unprotected sex (some rapists wear condoms to reduce the forensic evidence), you'll want advice on STDs and maybe emergency contraception. Hospitals and doctors are required to report the rape to the police, but it's up to you whether you want to press charges.
- If you decide to press charges, report what happened to the police as soon as possible. Medical evidence, if there is any, should ideally be collected within seventy-two hours of the attack.
- Don't wash or change your clothes, as you could destroy vital evidence. It's common to want to scrub yourself after an attack, so don't worry if you did this —you can still press charges.
- Take a change of clothes to the police station if you can, as the police might want to keep yours for evidence.
- It's your right to take a friend or relative for support, ask to see a female police officer, and be examined by a female doctor. You can leave the police station at any time if you feel uncomfortable.
- Don't feel under pressure to prosecute your attacker. It has to be your decision.

The identities of women who have been raped or sexually assaulted usually won't be revealed, so if you do press charges, there's a good chance that your name or photo won't be in the papers or on TV. You can report the crime to the police at any time, but it's best to report it sooner rather than later while there's still forensic evidence to collect. Rapists have been successfully convicted years after an attack, but such convictions are rare.

FEELINGS AFTER A SEXUAL ATTACK

With any rape or sexual assault, whatever the circumstances, the important thing to remember is that you're not responsible for what happened. Fear, shame, guilt, humiliation, and anger are common feelings after a sexual attack. You may get flashbacks of what happened and have nightmares, bouts of crying, or angry outbursts. You may not want anyone, particularly a man, near you. Such reactions are all perfectly normal, but don't feel you have to manage alone.

It will help you enormously to talk over what happened with a sympathetic friend, parent, teacher, or doctor, and you could also consider contacting a rape crisis center. The idea of calling one might be intimidating, but they really do understand the needs of girls and women who've suffered sexual attacks. Most offer free, confidential telephone or even face-to-face counseling, advice on what you can do about the attack, and general information. You can call the National Sexual Assault Hotline at 1-800-656-HOPE to find a counselor in your community. A call to a hotline is anonymous, as long as you don't reveal your name or phone number. For more specific help with the after-effects of abuse, see "Resources and Contacts."

Helping a Friend Who's Been Attacked

If someone you care about has suffered a sexual attack, you'll go through all kinds of emotions as you try to work out what's best to do. Perhaps you'll feel so upset and angry on your friend's behalf that you'll want to step in. Or at the other extreme, you may feel so helpless you can't think straight. Here are some ideas on how to help (and although I talk about "she" and "her," these would also apply to a male friend):

- *Ask what she needs from you.* You may have definite ideas as to what you'd like in her position, but don't assume she needs the same. She may want to curl up on your sofa and cry, go for a walk, or watch a DVD. Let her decide.
- *Give your friend space to process what happened to her.* She may want to go over and over the event with you, she may not want to talk about it at all, or she could be anywhere in between. She'll have her own personal response to the attack.
- *Don't impose your own judgments on her about the assault.* Perhaps she thought what happened was incredibly distressing and you thought it was pretty mild, or vice versa. She's entitled to her own feelings, whether you agree or not.
- *Protect her privacy.* It's tempting to confide in other friends and ask them what they think, but people talk and your friend will feel even more humiliated to discover that her ordeal has become gossip fodder. For advice, talk to an adult you trust or

contact an organization such as the National Sexual Assault Hotline at 1-800-656-HOPE. (See "Feelings After a Sexual Attack," page 236.)

- *Let your friend decide whether to report the attack.*
You may have strong feelings either way, but try to support your friend's decision. You can remind her gently that if she wants her attacker to be prosecuted, the crime needs to be reported as soon as possible, so the police can gather evidence. You or someone else can go with her to the police station if she wants.

STAYING SAFE

Although this chapter doesn't make for pleasant reading, it's vital to know the facts. Despite the acres of coverage they get in the media, violent crimes are actually pretty rare, thank goodness, and the good news is that there's a lot you can do to prevent yourself from becoming a victim.

Avoiding Drug Rape

* Of course, you shouldn't be drinking if you're under 21. But if you do, never leave your drink unattended, and take it to the bathroom with you. If you forget, leave it and buy another. *Any* drink can be spiked, not just alcoholic ones.

* Don't accept drinks from strangers, and if an acquaintance buys you a drink, make sure you see the bartender pour it. Then let the bartender hand it straight to you.

* If a group of you go out, designate one of you to keep an

eye on everyone's drinks. Don't share drinks or pick up discarded ones.

* Drink out of a bottle or can if possible, and keep your thumb over the opening. It's harder to drop drugs into bottles and cans.

Your drink may have been spiked if . . .

* You're drinking alcohol and feel weird, sick, or really drunk after a couple of sips.
* You're drinking soft drinks or tea, coffee, etc., and therefore can't possibly be drunk, but are feeling the above effects.

If you think your drink's been spiked . . .

* Get to a place of safety and tell a friend. Ask them to get you home as quickly as possible by taxi or car. You'll probably want them to call your parents.
* Make sure this is a person you know very well and trust completely.
* If you're alone or with a stranger, go to a senior staff member or the owner of wherever you are and tell them what's happened. Ask them to take you somewhere safe, like their office, while they contact your parents or a friend or get you a taxi.
* *Never* let a stranger take you home. He could be the rapist.

Keeping Safe While You're Out

* Plan the evening—where you're going, how you'll get there, how you'll get home.
* Always tell someone, such as your parents, where you're

going and when you'll be back. If your plans change, call or text and tell them the new time you'll be home.

* Be alert and aware of your surroundings when out and about.
* Trust your instincts—they're there to protect you.
* Walk confidently and keep to well-lit, busy roads. Avoid alleys and subways.
* Be careful when chatting on your cell phone or using anything with earphones—you might not hear someone approaching you from behind.
* Don't walk by yourself if possible—stick with friends.
* If you're out in a group, don't split up or leave someone to go home alone.
* On trains or buses, sit in a busy area or by the police officer or driver, and look around to locate the nearest alarm. If someone makes you feel uncomfortable, don't be embarrassed to move.
* If a car pulls up next to you, turn and run the opposite way. You can turn around quicker than a car.
* If you are followed, head into a store or toward people.
* Yell and make lots of noise to attract attention if someone threatens you. Run away if you can.
* Give away your purse, bag, or phone rather than fighting. Things can be replaced—you can't.

Safe Dates

* Arrange to meet in a busy place, preferably in the daytime, until you're sure the person is who they say they are and you're comfortable with them.
* If you barely know your date, take a friend along at first.

Arrange a signal to give your friend if you're happy for them to leave.

* Tell someone, preferably your parents, where you're going; the name, address, and phone number of the person you're meeting; and when you'll be back.

* Don't be completely alone with your date, go back to their place, or accept a ride until you know them well.

* Pay attention to your instincts. If you feel uneasy with your date, there's probably a good reason, even if you can't put your finger on it. Get away from them and don't see them again. You're not being paranoid—you're looking after yourself.

Net Know-How

* The Internet is fun and safe if you follow some simple rules. The biggie is never to give out personal details, such as your school, full name, address, phone number, or photo.

* Some adults will pretend to be kids and tell you what they think you want to hear so you'll trust them. Be aware that not everyone is who they say they are, however convincing they seem.

* If you find something that scares you online or receive nasty, pornographic, or threatening e-mails, tell an adult you trust.

* It's a very bad idea to meet up with anyone you've met online, as they could be dangerous. If you decide to go ahead, tell your parents what's happening, arrange to meet in a busy place, and take someone with you—an adult if possible. And don't forget your cell phone.

CHAPTER SEVENTEEN
Getting Pregnant

If you sleep with someone, you have to be prepared for the fact that you could become pregnant even if you're using contraception, because it can fail. There's only one way to ensure you don't get pregnant: don't have sex.

Other than genuine contraceptive failures, there might be the girl who decides that she probably can't conceive anyway and so isn't careful about contraception. Or the boy who won't wear condoms and says he'll pull out before he comes, but leaked sperm finds its way to the girl's womb and bang—a baby is begun. Or the girl who secretly wants a baby and regularly "forgets" to take her pills. Whatever and however, it's thought that as many as half of all pregnancies are unplanned. The United States has the highest teen pregnancy rate in the industrialized world. According to the National Campaign to Prevent Teen Pregnancy, 34 percent of American women become pregnant before the age of twenty. So sexually active teens are not being careful enough.

If you've had unprotected sex, don't forget that the emergency contraceptive pill taken within seventy-two hours or an IUD fitted within five days should prevent pregnancy. See chapter 10 for details.

This chapter is all about your choices if you do end up pregnant. It covers the following topics:

- Are You Pregnant?: If You're Not Pregnant...; If You're Pregnant...; Teenage Motherhood: The Reality
- Your Options: Keeping the Baby; Adoption; Abortion

ARE YOU PREGNANT?

You become pregnant when one of your eggs is fertilized by a boy's sperm and it successfully implants in the wall of your womb. It then starts to grow into a baby. A pregnancy is measured from the first day of your last period and normally lasts between thirty-seven and forty-two weeks (about nine months). About one in five pregnancies end in miscarriage, where the baby is lost. Most miscarriages happen in the first twelve weeks, and while some of these can be like a heavy period with lots of bleeding, other girls won't even realize they were ever pregnant.

Signs of pregnancy include:

- missing a period
- a period that's shorter or lighter than usual
- peeing frequently
- tiredness
- tender boobs
- nausea, vomiting (not necessarily in the morning), or abdominal cramps
- being repulsed by certain foods

If you've had sexual intercourse or sexual contact with a boy and get any of the above symptoms, you could be pregnant. The only way to find out for sure is to take a pregnancy test. If you are pregnant, the sooner you know the better. If you're going to continue with the pregnancy and either keep the baby or have it adopted, you need to arrange maternity (called pre-natal) care with a doctor to safeguard the health of yourself and the baby. Or if you choose to end the pregnancy, you need to act quickly. Pregnancy tests give you a result if taken any time from the first day of a missed period.

You can buy a home-testing kit for about thirteen dollars from a pharmacy or supermarket, and these are as reliable as tests done by a doctor. The advantage of these is that you get the results immediately and in complete privacy, although you might want a friend with you to discuss the result with. The test requires you to pee on a dipstick that changes color within a few minutes if you have traces of pregnancy hormone in your urine. Any change, however faint, means you're pregnant.

It's possible to get a negative (not pregnant) result that's wrong if your urine is very diluted, for example, if you've drunk a lot of liquid, or if the pregnancy hormone levels are very low. So if you get a negative result but your period hasn't come within three days, take another test.

False positives are rare, but you can sometimes get a positive (pregnant) result and then, days later, have your period. This may in fact be a very early miscarriage, but it doesn't mean you'll have problems getting pregnant in the future when you want a baby. Early miscarriage is very common, and is probably Nature's way of dealing with a baby that wouldn't have grown properly anyway.

If you go to a health clinic affiliated with Planned Parenthood for a pregnancy test, rest assured that it's all confidential and only you and the person who's testing you will be aware of what's going on. Generally there'll be a professional there for you to discuss the results with.

If You're Not Pregnant . . .

Heave a sigh of relief and go and talk to someone about either reviewing your contraception if it failed or getting contraception in place if you weren't using any. You might not be so lucky next time. Chapter 10 of this book discusses your contraceptive options in detail.

You can miss periods for various reasons (see chapter 2), but if you're worried about any symptoms, see your doctor.

If You're Pregnant . . .

Shock, fear, panic, loneliness, guilt, and confusion are common feelings on discovering you're pregnant. Then there's the huge worry about what your boyfriend will say and how your parents will react. At the same time many girls also find themselves feeling pleased that they can conceive. It's your pregnancy, and whatever you feel is OK.

As soon as you can, you need to decide what you're going to do: become a mother, have the baby and give it up for adoption, or end the pregnancy via abortion. Denial of the pregnancy and pretending the problem will go away if you act as though it's not happening is the worst thing you can do. If you're going to continue with the pregnancy you need medical care, and if you're going to have an abortion it needs to be arranged quickly.

Even if you're under sixteen, no one can force you to make a particular decision: it's your choice. And your choice may not be what your boyfriend or parents want.

What to do about an unplanned pregnancy is one of the most difficult decisions you will ever face, so please don't try to struggle with it on your own. You need support from those who love you and guidance from people who know the facts and can present them to you objectively. The first step is to tell someone. Your best friend, parents, and boyfriend will probably be first on the list.

It's true that parents can be very upset to discover that their daughter's pregnant, but after an initial outburst, most come around and offer support. They might want to visit http://www.kidshealth.org/parent/positive/talk/teen_pregnancy.html.

It's not an easy time, either, for the boy who fathered the baby. While some will want to share in any decisions, others won't want any involvement. Often they'll support what you want, even if it conflicts with their feelings. It's up to you whether you tell the father or not. Legally, the father has no right to be part of your final decision about the pregnancy, but it is his baby too, and that is something to consider.

While some girls know pretty much right away what they plan to do about the pregnancy, others feel so confused that it's hard to think logically about what would be best. That's why it's important to get the facts about *all* your options, but remember, the final choice is yours alone.

Teenage Motherhood: The Reality

A surprising number of young girls write to me saying they'd like to have a baby so they can have someone to themselves to love, who'll love them back. But romanticizing what it would be like to be a mother—that is, dwelling on the nice parts and ignoring the unpleasant ones—isn't helpful. Cuddly bundles soon become demanding toddlers needing all your attention. Having a baby puts an enormous strain on relationships, even among older couples who've been together many years and have plenty of money. And the fact is, teenage girls who have babies usually end up as one-parent families, because despite initial good intentions, many teenage dads can't cope with the pressure and leave. Nine out of ten teenage parents are very poor, living on welfare and in low-quality accommodations, with both mother and child's health often suffering as a result. And the children of teenage parents are themselves more likely to have kids in their teens.

YOUR OPTIONS

Keeping the Baby

If this is what you decide, see your family doctor or gynecologist, who will organize prenatal care. A large proportion of pregnant teenagers believe this is unnecessary and doesn't help much. In reality, not seeing a doctor or nurse for your regular health checks during pregnancy means you'll miss important tests for health problems such as diabetes and high blood pressure, which can affect the health of the mother and baby if not treated. You'll also need advice on what foods to eat and which to avoid, as some can harm the baby, and possibly to talk about cutting out or at least cutting down on cigarettes, alcohol, and other drugs.

Feelings About Keeping the Baby

There's no doubt that being a teenage mom is tough, and many say they wish they'd waited until they were older to have a baby. It can be difficult to complete your education, making it harder to climb out of the poverty trap, and it's easy to become isolated as your friends go out, have fun, and generally enjoy life without the major responsibility of bringing up a child. Never forget, though, that you have the same right as anyone else to respect and support for yourself and your baby, whatever your age.

On the positive side, you'll have tons of energy to run after and play with your little one, and you'll still be young when your child's grown up and left home. And you'll make new friends: other young moms like yourself who'll understand exactly what you're going through. Find them at your birthing class or ask your doctor or social worker about local teen mom support groups.

Adoption

Adoption provides your baby with new legal parents. Having a baby adopted is a lot less common today, as single parenthood has become more acceptable. If you think adoption might be for you, you'll still need to see your doctor to arrange for prenatal care throughout the pregnancy.

Adoptions can be arranged in three different ways: through a licensed government agency, through an independent adoption arranged by a private lawyer, and through an adoption by relatives arranged by the courts.

The National Adoption Information Clearinghouse can refer you to a licensed agency near you. You can call them at 1-888-251-0075. If you prefer an independent adoption, contact the Independent Adoption Center hotline at 1-800-877-6736. Each state has its own adoption laws.

There are so many people anxious to adopt that it should be no problem finding your baby a suitable, loving home. The agency or lawyer will want to hear the sort of family you'd like your child to be brought up in, and in an independent adoption you can probably meet the adoptive parents if you wish. Fathers' rights vary from state to state. Consult with a lawyer in your community to find out what your baby's father's involvement needs to be for an adoption to take place.

Giving up a baby that you carried through pregnancy and gave birth to is an enormous step that is never easy, and you have at least six weeks after the birth before you need to put your final agreement in writing. Once the adoption order has been through the courts, you'll no longer have any legal relationship with your child. However, you may be allowed to have some contact with him or her over the years if you've arranged for an independent, open adoption.

Feelings After the Adoption

Grief, loss, and anger mixed with feelings of relief are common after giving up a child for adoption. These might be immediate or may not crop up until long after the event, sometimes stirred up by other things that happen in your life. Sharing your feelings with someone sympathetic can help. If you can't talk to a friend or other trusted person, see "Resources and Contacts" for help.

Abortion

This is when the fetus (growing baby) is removed from the womb. It's done either by taking pills that will expel the pregnancy or by surgical procedures. Abortion arouses very strong feelings and can be hard to talk about. While some people think it's the woman's right to choose whether to have an abortion, others disagree. And a woman who agrees in principle that women should have the right to choose might still not feel that abortion is right for *her*.

Recent figures for the United States show that nearly one in three of all teen pregnancies end in abortion. Around nine out of ten abortions take place during the first twelve weeks of the pregnancy.

In the United States a girl or woman can have a safe, legal abortion in any state during her first trimester. Certain states limit access to abortions during the second trimester. Terminating a pregnancy after twenty-four weeks is very rare and can only take place if the mother's life is in danger or if there's something seriously wrong with the fetus. At the time of writing, new information has come to light about a baby's development in the womb, and there are attempts being made to reduce the number of weeks into a pregnancy an abortion can be performed.

If, after careful thought and discussion with sympathetic people who understand all the options available, a woman decides she wants to end her pregnancy, she will need to see a doctor.

Most abortions are performed because (a) having the baby would harm the woman's mental or physical health more than an abortion—for example, if going ahead with the pregnancy would make her very distressed or depressed; or (b) there's a substantial risk that the baby would be born severely disabled.

There are other reasons—for example, if continuing the pregnancy would risk the woman's life—but most abortions are performed because the woman falls into the first category.

Legally, the father of the baby doesn't need to agree to or even be told about the abortion, although it's usually better for both of you if he's involved, if possible.

Underage Abortions

Each state has its own laws regarding a teen's right to an abortion without notifying a parent. Call Planned Parenthood at 1-800-230-PLAN to find out about parental notification laws in your state, and to locate a health clinic that will perform an abortion.

You can also check with your family doctor or gynecologist to see if they perform abortions.

Abortion is a serious matter for which a girl will need emotional support and possibly physical care afterward, so it's best for her to involve her parents if she can.

What Does It Involve?

There are different methods of terminating a pregnancy, depending on how many weeks pregnant a woman is. Depending on the stage of pregnancy, she generally has some say in the kind of procedure she will undergo. Abortion is simpler in the early stages of pregnancy, which is why it's best to arrange it as soon as possible.

Feelings After an Abortion

Any combination of feelings after an abortion are normal, and no two women will react in exactly the same way. Relief at having dealt with the pregnancy is common, along with the feeling of having made the best choice she could in a difficult situation. She might also feel sad, depressed, or guilty, and need to grieve the loss. Some women might not feel much immediately after the procedure, but weeks, months, or years later, feelings about the abortion may crop up.

Talking to a friend, relative, or other person she trusts can help a girl sort out her feelings. If that's not appropriate, she could see a professional counselor. There's a list of organizations that can help in "Resources and Contacts."

CHAPTER EIGHTEEN

Your Most Embarrassing Sex Questions Answered

In this last chapter, I've put together questions that might crop up when talking to your friends or boyfriend, or from watching TV programs or reading magazines, and that you can't quite bring yourself to ask. So if you have any questions left (*phew!*), hopefully you'll find the answers here. This chapter covers:

- What's a blow job?
- How long does sex take?
- What's 69?
- What's a vibrator?
- Can we stop my boyfriend from coming so quickly?
- What positions can you have sex in?
- Why do people have anal sex?
- How do lesbians have sex?
- What happens in a threesome?
- What if I do sex wrong?

What's a blow job?

My boyfriend has asked me to give him a blow job, but I'm not sure what's involved. Can it make me pregnant?

A blow job is another term for performing oral sex on a boy (using your mouth and tongue on his penis). The name is misleading, as you should never blow into a penis. Oral sex is an extremely intimate act that not everyone is comfortable with, so, like all sexual activities, you have a right to say no if you don't want to do this. If you choose to go ahead, experts say a condom should be used to avoid passing on STDs, but if you and your partner have been tested for STDs at a clinic and found to be clear, you could do it without. Many girls prefer to take their mouth away before the boy ejaculates (comes); others discreetly spit the semen into a tissue. Swallowing semen can't get you pregnant. For there to be a chance of pregnancy, the semen has to go up the girl's vagina to her womb.

How long does sex take?

How long should the actual banging part of sex go on for? And how does the penis get into the vagina? Does the guy put it there or does it find its own way in?

The penis needs help to enter the vagina, so it can be the boy, the girl, or both together who guide it in by hand. Before this happens, it's nice to have what's known as foreplay, where both partners stroke and kiss each other. This helps the girl's vagina to relax and start producing the clear fluid that lubricates the area so the penis can go in easily. If a girl is tense or dry down below, sex can be difficult or even impossible. Once the penis is inside, the boy moves in and out until he ejaculates (comes), which can take anywhere from a few seconds to half an hour or so. But rather than using a stopwatch, it's better for both partners to let their feelings gauge how long each stage takes.

What's 69?

I've heard people talk about a sexual position called 69. What is it?

This is where two people perform oral sex on each other at the same time. It's called 69 because of the way the two bodies are arranged, with a head at either end. For safe oral sex, use a condom on the boy and a latex square (also called a dental dam) on the girl (see chapter 11, "Sexually Transmitted Diseases and Women's Health"), unless both have been tested for STDs and found to be clear. In practice, it's not easy to find a comfortable position for this, plus there's so much going on that it can be difficult to concentrate on either giving or receiving pleasure.

What's a vibrator?

My friend says her mom has a vibrator in her drawer. What are these used for and where can you get them?

Vibrators are plastic devices, often but not always penis shaped, that are battery operated and vibrate like crazy when switched on. Contrary to popular belief, women don't tend to put them up their vagina. Rather, they're held against the clitoris to give a woman an orgasm. Sex therapists sometimes recommend these to women who can't have an orgasm by the usual means. Then once she's learned what an orgasm feels like, she can discover how to give one to herself without the vibrator and pass this information on to her partner. Women might also keep a vibrator to masturbate with or to use with a partner.

Can we stop my boyfriend from coming so quickly?

When we have sex, my boyfriend often comes almost immediately. This doesn't particularly bother me, but he's upset about it. What can we do?

This is known as premature ejaculation and it's very common, particularly in young men. Sometimes a boy gets so excited at the prospect of sex that he just can't help coming before he wants to. But as he gets used to being in a relationship, having sex, and the reactions of his own body, this tends to happen less and he gains more control. Condoms, which you should use anyway to stave off pregnancy and STDs, can reduce sensation and make premature ejaculation less of a problem.

What positions can you have sex in?

My friend says there are hundreds of positions that you can have sex in, but I'm not so sure. How many are there?

Some books suggest lots of different positions, but it's pointless struggling into some complicated position just to prove how athletic you are if the end result is a cramp or a stiff neck. The most popular positions for sex are face to face, so you can communicate with your partner and watch their reactions. So the missionary position, with the boy on top and girl underneath, is probably the most popular, closely followed by the boy underneath and the girl on top. Other common ones are "doggy style," where the girl kneels on all fours with the boy behind her, and "spoons," in which you both lie on your side curved against one another with the girl in front. Sex standing up is practically impossible unless the boy is strong enough to lift and hold the girl up, which few are. What matters is that both partners are enjoying themselves and are protected against pregnancy and STDs, so it's up to them to use their imagination and see what they come up with.

Why do people have anal sex?

I've heard that some people have anal sex. Why would they do this?

Anal sex is where a boy puts his penis in the anus (rectal opening) of another person. The anus has a lot of nerve endings, so some people find this pleasurable, but it can also be very painful because the rectum isn't as elastic as the vagina. Anal sex is the riskiest kind of sex for passing on sexually transmitted diseases because the inside of the back passage is tight, and the delicate skin can tear easily. Many people don't like anal sex, but for those who do, condoms must always be used to protect against diseases. And like all forms of sexual contact, don't forget it's your right to refuse if your boyfriend suggests this and you don't want to try it.

How do lesbians have sex?
What do lesbians do in bed? I just can't imagine what two women would do together.

Lesbians make love to each other using their hands and mouths. They enjoy similar things to boys and girls during foreplay that you don't need a penis for—kissing, stroking, touching, etc. Breasts usually play a large part, as obviously both partners have them. It's often assumed that lesbians copy heterosexual (male-female) sex and use penis-shaped objects (dildos) on each other. Some use these, but others don't like them—as with all couples, what goes on depends on the individuals involved.

What happens in a threesome?
My boyfriend keeps dropping hints about me having sex with him and his best friend. I don't think I want to, but how would it work?

A threesome is when three people do whatever sexual stuff they like to each other—there's no set way of going about it. It's true that a few people think a threesome sounds like a great idea and try to bring a third party into the relationship, like your boyfriend is hinting at. However, the relationships can then fall apart because those involved get jealous and/or feel used. I'd be very worried about a boy who thinks it's OK to suggest this. You're not a toy for him to pass between his friends. No boy who cared for and respected his girlfriend would dream of pressuring her into sleeping with him and his friend. And it's a good way to catch a disease or get pregnant because people who have that little respect for others don't care what they're passing on.

What if I do sex wrong?

I've never slept with anyone and I'm worried that I'll do it wrong and the boy will laugh. Do you have any tips?

Sex isn't something you pass or fail, like an exam. Ideally, the desire to have sex grows out of the deep feelings you and your partner have for each other. That means that you know each other well enough to be able to laugh together when something funny happens—and, believe me, it will. Stomachs rumble, people fall off beds, condoms shoot across the room when you're trying to get them on, the odd fart will ring out—in fact, it's pretty common for the vagina to make a farting noise when the penis slides out during sex. (Remedy that one by making sure you've been kissing and cuddling long enough for your vagina to become lubricated.) It's true that sex in the abstract is scary, but when you're learning the ropes alongside someone you trust completely, are crazy about the person, and are using contraception, it's a fun and exciting voyage of discovery. So don't worry. It will be fine if you wait for the right boy and until you feel completely ready.

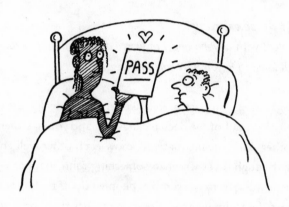

RESOURCES AND CONTACTS

If you have questions or a problem, there are lots of organizations that can help. Here's a selection, most of which have been mentioned in the book. Before calling, it's a good idea to have a pen and paper handy.

Adoption

Adopting.org
http://www.adopting.org
1-800-537-2229

Adopting.org has easy-to-access information for those considering adoption services, including those who wish to take in a child and those who wish to place a child. The site includes advice for adoptive parents and support for birth parents and families. There are local addresses available on the Web site, but here's the information for the New York office.

LDS Family Services
NY New York Agency
One Civic Center Plaza, Suite 530
Poughkeepsie, NY 12601-3460
PH: 845-462-1288
FAX: 845-462-1291

Bullying

National Crime Prevention Council (NCPC)
http://www.ncpc.org

NCPC is a nonprofit organization whose mission is to prevent crime and build safer, more caring communities. It includes informational reading material, brochures, educational resources, and "McGruff the Crime Dog" videos and activities. This is more helpful to adults trying to find out how to keep kids safe or educate teens.

National Youth Violence Prevention Resource Center
http://www.safeyouth.org/scripts/contactform.asp
1-866-SAFEYOUTH (1-866-723-3968)
1-888-503-3952 (TTY)

This site provides a help line and pamphlets for all levels of teen abuse, as well as a list of sites according to issue, including juveniles in adult court, anxiety disorders, after-school programs, and bullying.

Stop Bullying Now!
http://www.stopbullyingnow.hrsa.gov/
comments@hrsa.gov

Stop Bullying Now! is a Web site built by and for kids and teens. It's very accessible for young children and includes information on how to recognize bullying and take measures to stay safe. You can e-mail them for pamphlets or more information.

Tolerance.org
http://www.tolerance.org
334-956-8200

Tolerance.org encourages people from all walks of life to work to eliminate hatred and promote tolerance. They promote community or group-oriented action.

Drugs and Alcohol

Alcoholics Anonymous (AA)

http://www.alcoholics-anonymous.org

AA's primary purpose is to assist alcoholics in recovery. AA also lists symptoms of specific drugs and offers pamphlets on sobriety and drinking. There is a special section for teens, which includes helpful ways of knowing when drinking is a problem.

American Council for Drug Education

http://www.acde.org

The ACDE is a prevention and education agency against substance abuse. This Web site includes a helpful list of symptoms associated with specific drugs. It includes a discussion list for those who wish to join an online support community.

Drughelp.org

http://www.drughelp.org

DrugHelp is a private nonprofit information and referral network providing information on specific drugs and treatment options and referrals to public and private treatment programs, self-help groups, family support groups, and crisis centers throughout the United States.

Narcotics Anonymous (NA)

http://www.wsoinc.com
818-773-9999

NA is an international, community-based association of recovering drug addicts.

Eating Disorders

ANRED: Anorexia Nervosa and Related Eating Disorders
http://www.anred.com

ANRED is a nonprofit organization with information about eating disorders. ANRED offers material that stresses recovery and prevention of eating disorders. They include an e-mail address for questions not addressed on their site.

Center for Eating Disorders
http://www.eating-disorders.com
410-427-2100

St. Joseph Medical Center's Center for Eating Disorders offers news, information, and support.

National Eating Disorder Association (NEDA)
http://www.nationaleatingdisorders.org
Toll-free Information and Referral Helpline: 1-800-931-2237

NEDA is the largest nonprofit organization in the United States working to prevent eating disorders and provide treatment referrals to those suffering from anorexia, bulimia, and binge eating disorder, and those concerned with body image and weight issues.

Overeaters Anonymous
http://www.overeatersanonymous.org

This organization is dedicated to helping people recover from compulsive overeating.

Gay and Lesbian Issues

AVERT
http://www.avert.org/gaylesbianhelp.htm

AVERT is an international AIDS charity that also provides a list of resources for those who are lesbian, gay, bisexual, or uncertain of their sexual orientation.

The Gay and Lesbian National Hotline
www.glnh.org/home.htm
1-800-246-PRIDE (youth hotline)
1-888-THE-GLNH (gay & lesbian national hotline)

The Gay, Lesbian, Bisexual, Transgendered (GLBT) National Help Center provides free and confidential telephone and e-mail peer counseling, information, and local resources for those who question their sexuality or need a supportive site on being gay, lesbian, bisexual, or transgendered. Peer counselors are available Monday through Friday, from 4:00 p.m. to midnight, and Saturday from noon to 5:00 p.m. EST.

National Gay and Lesbian Youth Hotline
1-800-347-TEEN (weekend nights only)

National Gay and Lesbian Youth Hotline is a weekend support line for youth in crisis.

QueerAmerica
http://www.queeramerica.com

QueerAmerica is a database that searches local resources, support organizations, and community centers based on your area code and zip code.

Life Problems/General

4Girls
http://www.4girls.gov

4Girls, developed by the U.S. Office on Women's Health, offers girls between the ages of ten and sixteen information about growing up, food and fitness, and relationships. It also includes information and references to other sites on all issues for girls, including pregnancy.

American Psychological Association (APA)
http://www.apa.org

The APA provides information and education about a variety of mental health issues for people of all ages.

TeensHealth
http://kidshealth.org/teen/

This is a great resource, with all the information you need as a teen, from when you're ready for body piercing to when you're ready for sex, from tips on healthy food to drug abuse, from how to deal with bug bites to how to deal with assaults. The information on their site is very accessible and includes articles, quizzes, personal testimonies, a list of resources, and a simple breakdown for each category. Although TeenHealth doesn't have a hotline number, they do provide a listing of hotline numbers for other organizations.

Parenting

Advocates for Youth's My Voice Counts Youth Action Center
http://www.advocatesforyouth.org/youth/

This site provides general information on adolescent sexual and reproductive health and information on what you can do to make a difference.

National Campaign to Prevent Teen Pregnancy
http://www.teenpregnancy.org/teen

This site provides teen pregnancy facts, resources, and prevention tips for parents and teens.

Sex, Etc.
http://www.sexetc.org

By teens for teens, this site helps youth become sexually healthy people and avoid pregnancy and disease during their teenage years.

Personal Safety

Cyberangels
http://www.cyberangels.org

Cyberangels.org is an Internet safety organization that seeks to address the concerns of parents, the needs of children, online abuse, and cyber crime.

Join Together
http://www.jointogether.org
617-437-1500

Join Together, a project of the Boston University School of Public Health, is a national resource for communities working to reduce substance abuse and gun violence.

National Center for Victims of Crime
http://www.ncvc.org
1-800-FYI-CALL (1-800-211-7996)

This organization is devoted to helping victims of crime recover and rebuild their lives.

The Rape, Abuse & Incest National Network
http://www.rainn.org
1-800-656-HOPE

This is a nationwide network of more than 1,100 local rape treatment hotlines that provide victims of sexual assault with confidential treatment around the clock.

SafeTeens.com
http://www.safeteens.com

SafeTeens.com offers information about Internet safety as well as homework help for teens.

Sexual Health/Contraception/Unplanned Pregnancy

American Social Health Association
http://www.iwannaknow.org
http://www.ashastd.org

STI Resource Center: 1-800-227-8922

This site is a good source of information about preventing and treating STDs. They also have tips for reducing risk and suggestions for talking to health care providers and sexual partners.

Centers for Disease Control and Prevention (CDC)

http://www.cdcnpin.org/scripts/index.asp

National STD Hotline at 1-800-227-8922 or 1-800-342-2437

Prevention Information Network at 1-800-458-5231

Prevention e-mail: info@cdcnpin.org

Prevention mailing address:

CDC NPIN

P.O. Box 6003

Rockville, MD 20849-6003

The Centers for Disease Control and Prevention (CDC) is a great site for gathering information through their Web pages, pamphlets, and database of organizations. They also have a national hotline number for asking questions.

Planned Parenthood Federation of America

http://www.plannedparenthood.org

1-800-230-PLAN (1-800-230-7526)

http://www.teenwire.com

This site from the Planned Parenthood Federation of America has information on relationships and sexual health for teens. It also includes referrals to local clinics.

ACKNOWLEDGMENTS

Thanks to everyone who helped with information for this book, with particular mention to:

Kerry Parnell, who wrote the original book this edition is based on and who provided three of the quizzes; Rebecca Findlay of the fpa, whose leaflets provided most of the information on contraception, STDs, and abortion; The Eating Disorders Association for facts and figures on eating disorders plus tips on improving self-esteem; the Suzy Lamplugh Trust for information on personal safety from their guidance sheets; Dr. Helen Jones of Manchester Metropolitan University and Clare Hoban of Emap for legal advice; the Roofie Foundation for advice on drugs used in rape and sexual assaults, and avoiding drug-assisted attacks; The Truth About Rape campaign for information on rape, rape crisis services, and what to do after a sexual attack; Brook Advisory Centres; Dr. Christiane Northrup; Marian Nicholson of the Herpes Association; The British Association of Adoption and Fostering (BAAF); Teenage Pregnancy Advisor Anne Patterson; The Citizenship Foundation; Chris Baxter; Dr. Denise Syndercombe Court. Thanks also to my editor at Piccadilly, Yasemin Uçar, and the staff of *bliss* magazine.

INDEX

abortion, 152, 207, 242, 245, 249–51
abuse, 94, 123, 224, 226–29, 236,
    260, 266 (*see also* incest)
acne, 3, 8, 15, 28, 137, 140, 143, 148 (*see also* skin)
addiction, 111–112
adolescence, 4, 180–82 (*see also* puberty)
adopting.org, 259
adoption, 242, 243, 245, 248–49, 259
Advocates for Youth's My Voice
    Counts Youth Action Center, 265
affirmations, 54–55
age of consent, 84, 101–2, 105–6, 116,
    119, 200, 229 (*see also* consent; laws)
ageofconsent.com, 102
AIDS, 125, 146, 157, 167–68, 207, 263
alcohol
    abuse of, 228, 261
    antibiotics and, 173, 174
    sex and, 76, 117, 123, 220, 223
    sexual assaults and, 224, 231, 233,
        234, 238
Alcoholics Anonymous (AA), 261
American Council for Drug
    Education, 261
American Psychological Association
    (APA), 264
American Social Health Association,
    163, 266
anal sex, 252, 255–56
anemia, 27
anorexia nervosa, 36, 41–42, 262
ANRED: Anorexia Nervosa and
    Related Eating Disorders, 262
antibiotics, 58
    contraceptives and, 137, 142, 147,
        149
    for STDs, 161, 164, 166, 169,
        172, 173, 175, 176, 178
antiperspirants, 9, 16 (*see also*
    deodorants)
appearance, 36–42, 49–53, 68–71,
    86–87, 95, 99, 180, 186, 218, 222
    (*see also* body image)
    changes in, 6, 15
arousal, sexual, 11–14, 85, 121, 220, 254
    (*see also* foreplay; masturbation)
attitudes, 69, 95–104 (*see also* values)
attraction, 68–75, 82, 86–87, 92–93, 182
AVERT, 263

bacteria, friendly, 12, 128, 175, 176
bacterial vaginosis (BV), 157, 174–75
balls (*see* testicles)

binge-eating, 42, 43, 262
birth control (*see* contraception)
bisexuality, 93, 263–64
bleeding (*see* periods; vagina, bleeding
    from)
blow job, 201, 216, 252–53
blue balls, 20, 188–89 (*see also* testicles)
body, changes in, 4–24, 63, 180
body hair, 7–9, 11, 15, 62–63, 150, 169–70
    (*see also* hair)
body image, 6, 36–40, 50–53, 99,
    180–81, 262 (*see also* appearance;
    self-esteem)
body language, 68, 69–70, 205
body size and shape, 3, 4, 6, 15, 37–38,
    41, 43, 45, 50, 63, 180 (*see also*
    height; weight)
boob jobs, 36, 46, 48–50, 52 (*see also*
    breasts)
boyfriends, 58, 85, 92, 106–12, 216,
    252–53
    dating, 67, 77–83
    porn and, 103, 105, 111–12, 225
    pregnancy and, 245–46, 250
    pressure from, 100, 117, 120, 184,
        187–191, 224, 231–32, 256–57
    talking with, 181, 192–93, 199–205,
        214, 219–21, 252
boys, 44, 45, 51, 57, 73, 76–77, 86–87,
    93, 112, 231
    attracting, 3, 67–75, 76–77
    contraception for, 129–35
    masturbation by, 90–91
    physical changes in, 4, 6, 8, 14,
        15–20
    sex and, 100, 111–12, 116, 117,
        180–92, 197, 201, 213, 215–19,
        221–23, 225, 252–55
    STDs in, 158, 161, 163, 164, 166,
        169, 173, 177
bras, 36, 44, 45, 47, 48, 50, 62
breaking up, 82–83
breasts, 4–6, 13, 36, 44–50, 85, 167, 171
    (*see also* boob jobs; cancer, breast)
    size of, 17, 37, 45–46, 57, 62, 180
    soreness in, 25, 28, 138, 140, 143,
        150, 153, 243 (*see also*
        symptoms)
    touching, 73–74, 91, 256
bulimia nervosa, 36, 41, 42, 262
bullying, 57, 100, 187, 225, 259–60 (*see
    also* teasing)

calcium, 27, 29

cancer
 breast, 47–48, 62, 138, 150 (*see also* breasts)
 cervical, 59, 138, 145, 160, 165 (*see also* cervix)
 ovarian, 137
 uterine, 137 (*see also* womb)
candida (*see* yeast infections)
caps, 125, 130, 144–46, 209
CDC (Centers for Disease Control and Prevention), 267
cellulite, 57, 59–60
Center for Eating Disorders, 262
cervical smear, 59, 165
cervix, 12, 21–24, 59, 60, 128, 162, 176 (*see also* cancer, cervical; mucus, cervical; womb)
chat rooms, 88, 241 (*see also* Internet)
Childhelp USA, 228
chlamydia, 157, 158, 160–61, 165, 176
circumcision, 18
clinics, 31, 59, 120, 193, 200, 206–11, 244, 250, 267
 contraception from, 125, 126–27, 135, 139, 146, 149, 151, 154, 155
 STDs treated at, 156–58, 159, 160
clitoris, 10, 11, 17, 85–86, 201, 212
 stimulation of, 14, 90, 91, 215, 222, 254
cold sores (*see* herpes, facial and genital)
combination pill (*see* contraceptive pill)
comfort-eating, 42
coming (*see* ejaculation; orgasms)
communication (*see* fights; talking about sex)
complexion (*see* acne; skin)
condoms, 58, 199, 201, 205, 211, 212, 216, 235, 255, 256, 257
 for contraception, 129, 130–35, 136, 137, 138, 139, 140, 141, 143, 146, 147, 148, 149, 150, 151
 failure of, 242
 female, 131, 132–33, 134–35, 211, 254
 for STD protection, 156, 161, 163, 166, 167–69, 172, 173, 174, 175, 177
confidence, 49, 52, 77, 120, 180, 183, 190, 201, 202, 213, 220, 225, 240 (*see also* self-esteem)
confidentiality, 126, 157, 159, 193, 207–09, 236, 244, 263
consent (*see also* age of consent)
 to contraception, 193, 207
 for marriage, 109
 to sex, 101–02, 227, 229–30, 231

contraception, 115, 116, 117, 120, 125–55, 200, 207–13, 216, 220, 257 (*see also* pregnancy)
 emergency, 125, 130, 152–55, 212, 235, 242
 failure of, 31, 220, 242, 244
 resources for, 267
contraceptive injection, 125, 130, 141–43
contraceptive patch, 125, 130, 149–51
contraceptive pill, 12, 27, 30, 58, 130, 207
 combination pill, 125, 130, 136–39, 141, 142, 150, 178–79
 emergency pill, 152–55, 212
 forgetting to take, 242
 progestin-only pill (POP or Mini-Pill), 125, 130, 138–40, 143, 145, 146
cosmetic surgery, 37, 46, 48–50, 52, 99
counseling/counselors, 82, 93, 196, 207, 208, 209, 228, 236, 251
crabs (*see* pubic lice)
cramps, 26–27, 243
crushes, 4, 79, 86, 110 (*see also* love)
culture, 69, 98, 109, 118, 121
cunnilingus, 201
Cyberangels, 265
cybersex, 88
cystitis, 145, 157, 175–76

date rape, 224, 231–34, 238–39
dating/dates, 67–83, 103, 105, 107, 112, 180, 189, 192, 229
 first, 5, 67
 safe, 224, 240–41
deodorants, 9, 16, 174, 178 (*see also* antiperspirants)
Depo-Provera, 141, 142
depression, 28, 30, 41, 143, 210, 225, 228, 250, 251
diaphragms, 125, 130, 144–46, 209
diet, 8, 26–27, 29, 40, 52, 59, 64, 247
dieting, 30, 38–43, 50–52, 63–64, 99
discharge, 25, 47, 58, 158, 160–61, 165, 169, 173, 174, 177, 209
doctors, 8, 12, 26, 27, 43, 59, 218, 232, 235, 236
 contraception from, 120, 126, 127, 137, 138, 139, 142, 146, 148, 149, 151, 155, 156, 200, 211
 pregnancy help from, 243, 244, 247, 248, 250
 STD treatment from, 58, 156–57, 158, 160, 161, 164, 165, 166, 167, 168, 169, 170, 171, 172, 173, 174, 175, 176, 178
 talking with, 30, 47, 193, 196, 200, 206–210
double standards, 183–84

dreams, 89 (*see also* wet dreams)
drinking (*see* alcohol)
Drughelp.org, 261
drug rape, 223, 233–34, 238–39
drugs
    abuse of, 167, 196, 210, 228, 247, 261–62
    antidepressant, 30
    anti-viral, 163
    date-rape, 224, 233–34, 238–39 (*see also* GHB; Rohypnol)
    epilepsy, 149
    sex and, 123, 223, 231
dyke, 186

eating disorders, 36, 41–43, 228, 262–63
ectopic pregnancy, 154
eggs, release of, 23–25, 136, 139, 141, 147, 149, 152
ejaculation, 14, 17, 19–20, 91, 116, 127, 131, 188–89, 217, 254–55 (*see also* pre-ejaculate; premature ejaculation)
emergency contraception, 125, 130, 151–55, 212, 235, 242
emotions, 27, 30, 54–56, 67, 77, 105–12, 123, 181, 185, 186, 191
    about abortion, 249, 251
    after rape, 236
    sexual, 4, 5, 84, 89, 92, 102, 120–21, 219–21
epididymis, 19
erections, 17–20, 127–28, 132, 133, 182, 188, 211–12, 215–16, 223
estrogen (*see* hormones)
ex-boyfriends, 83, 231
exercise, 26, 29, 39, 40, 42, 59, 63–64, 116, 223

faces, changes in, 6, 15, 37
facial hair, 15, 62–63
Fallopian tubes, 21, 22, 24, 160, 176–77
fantasies, 86, 87, 110
fathers, rights of, 246, 248, 250
feelings (*see* emotions)
fellatio, 201
female condoms (*see* condoms)
fertility, 24, 126, 128, 143, 159, 160, 177
fertilization, 24, 136, 147, 152, 155, 243
fetus, 249
fights, 4, 79–80
fingers, 157, 161–62, 164
first-time sex, 5, 13, 59, 116–18, 187, 190, 204, 211–213, 217–21 (*see also* sexual intercourse)
flashers, 224, 226
foreplay, 214–16, 218, 221, 253, 256 (*see also* stimulation, sexual)

foreskin, 18, 177 (*see also* skin)
4Girls, 264
friends, 3, 4, 5, 40, 45, 50, 52, 68, 69, 72, 73, 74, 75, 77, 80, 90, 94, 100–101, 104, 107, 109–10, 111, 112, 181, 184, 208, 218, 219, 256–57
    pregnancy and, 245, 247, 249
    pressure from, 106, 120, 184, 185, 190, 204–05, 213
    rape and, 224, 228, 232, 234, 237–38
    safety with, 238, 239
    talking with, 55, 83, 87–88, 98, 193, 197–99, 202, 251, 252
frigid, 185, 191

gays (*see* homosexuals)
Gay and Lesbian National Hotline, The 263
Gay, Lesbian, Bisexual, Transgendered (GLBT) National Help Center, 263
genitals, 97, 157, 169, 199, 200, 209, 226
    female, 9–13, 34, 133
    male, 16, 17–20, 132
    odor of, 57–58
    soreness in, 58, 158, 161, 162–64, 169–70, 172, 173, 176, 218, 222, 233, 253 (*see also* symptoms)
    stimulation of, 84, 88, 89–90, 214–16
genital warts, 158, 163–65
GHB, 233 (*see also* drugs, date-rape)
girls
    differences from boys, 180–82
    masturbation by, 91
    physical changes in, 5–14, 63
gonorrhea, 157, 158, 165–66, 173, 176, 210
GPs (*see* doctors)
G-spot, 12–13, 14
guilt, 156, 188, 251 (*see also* regrets)

hair, 4, 8, 15, 36, 37, 41, 51, 52, 69, 70, 71, 169–70 (*see also* body hair; pubic hair; shaving)
healthy eating (*see* diet)
height, 4, 6, 15, 180 (*see also* body size and shape)
help lines, 137, 138, 163, 193, 208, 210, 228, 259–67
hepatitis B, 157, 166
herpes, facial and genital, 157, 161–63, 210
heterosexuals, 92–93
HIV, 125, 146, 157, 167–69, 207, 210, 211
homophobia, 85, 93–94, 184
homosexuals, 85, 92–94, 96, 103, 109–10, 167, 184, 263–64 (*see also* lesbians; sexual orientation)

hormones, 5, 8, 17–18, 47, 59, 84, 85, 147, 244
    balance of, 25–30, 130
    estrogen, 5, 23, 136, 140, 141, 149
    progesterone, 5, 23, 136, 139, 141
    progestin, 139, 146, 147, 149, 152
    testosterone, 8, 15, 23, 181–82
hotlines, 193, 236, 259–67
hygiene, 8–9, 16, 18, 58, 71
hymen, 13, 35, 116, 211, 217

incest, 266 (see also abuse)
Independent Adoption Center, 248
intercourse (see sexual intercourse)
Internet, 88, 98, 103, 241, 265–66 (see also chat rooms)
intimacy, 87, 120, 204–05
intrauterine devices (IUD and IUS), 130, 146–47, 151, 209
    as emergency contraception, 155, 242
iron, 27

jaundice, 166
jealousy, 50, 67, 80–81, 189, 257
Join Together, 265–66

kidshealth.org, 246, 264–65
kissing, 68, 72, 86, 87, 103, 119, 167, 203, 211, 214, 215, 221, 253, 256, 257
    first, 3, 5
    French, 215

labia, 10, 11
lactobacillus acidophilus (see bacteria, friendly)
latex squares, 161, 166, 167, 169, 173, 254
laws, 96, 101–03, 105, 109, 205
    (see also age of consent)
    abortion, 250
    adoption, 248–49
    sexual assault, 224, 228–29, 234–35, 238
LDS Family Services, 259
lesbians, 86–87, 102, 109–10, 186, 256, 263–64 (see also homosexuals)
looks (see appearance)
love, 78–79, 117, 118, 187–88, 191, 219 (see also crushes)
Lunelle, 141, 143
lying, 188, 191

magnesium, 27, 29
masturbation, 84–85, 87, 88, 89–92, 111, 182, 212, 254 (see also arousal, sexual; stimulation, sexual)
maturity, 106, 111, 116, 119, 181

media, 36–38, 94, 95, 99, 101, 104, 184, 219, 238
menstruation (see periods)
mental health, 41, 46, 250
Mini-Pill (see contraceptive pill)
miscarriages, 243–44
missionary position, 217, 255
mons pubis, 10
morning-after pills (see emergency contraception)
mucus, cervical, 12, 23–24, 136, 139, 141, 147, 149 (see also cervix)
myths
    about masturbation, 85, 90–91
    about pregnancy, 125, 127–28
    about rape, 230–31
    about sex, 69, 214, 222–23

name-calling, 94, 185–87, 191, 225
Narcotics Anonymous (NA), 261–62
National Adoption Information Clearinghouse, 248
National Campaign to Prevent Teen Pregnancy, 265
National Center for Victims of Crime, 230, 266
National Crime Prevention Council (NCPC), 259–60
National Eating Disorder Association (NEDA), 262
National Gay and Lesbian Youth Hotline, 93, 263
National Sexual Assault Hotline, 236, 238
National U.S. Herpes Hotline, 163
National Youth Violence Prevention Resource Center, 225, 260
natural family planning, 125, 128
nipples, 6–7, 13, 20, 36, 44–50, 62
non-specific genital infections (NSGIs), 157, 169
nutrition (see diet)
nymphomaniac, 186, 201

oils, skin, 8, 15
one-parent families (see single parents)
oral sex, 135, 158, 160, 161–162, 166, 169, 173, 201, 211–12, 214, 216, 252–54 (see also "69")
orgasms, 3, 11, 13–14, 20, 88, 89, 91, 92, 127, 214, 216–17, 221, 254
os, 12
ovaries, 21, 22–23, 137, 140, 148
Overeaters Anonymous, 262
ovulation, 21, 23–24, 25, 127

pads, 21, 27, 31–33, 35, 60, 178

pain, 49, 63 (*see also* symptoms)
  abdominal, 153, 154, 160, 165, 175, 176
  during periods, 21, 26–30, 34–35, 137, 140, 148, 150
  during sex, 158, 161, 173, 177, 205, 217, 255–56
  during urination, 58, 158, 160–61, 162, 165, 169, 173, 175, 177
  in genital area, 141, 158, 161, 162, 177
  pelvic, 137, 141
panty liners, 33, 178
pap smear (*see* cervical smear)
parenting, 264
parents, 4, 5, 76, 95, 101, 108–09, 121, 179, 206–07, 219, 225, 239
  pregnancy and, 245–46
  talking with, 96–97, 193–96
pedophiles, 93–94
peeing (*see* urination)
peer pressure, 100, 106, 180, 193, 197–99 (*see also* pressure to have sex)
pelvic inflammatory disease (PID), 142, 157, 160, 176–77
penis, 11–20, 85, 127, 131, 133, 161–68, 189, 201, 226, 252–55
  discharge from, 158, 161, 173
  insertion of, 35, 84, 116, 134, 217, 253
  size of, 180, 222–23
  stimulation of, 91, 215–16, 221
periods, 5, 13, 21–35, 41, 43, 47, 60–61, 85, 118, 142–43, 148–50, 153–54, 155, 163, 167
  bleeding between, 138, 140, 141, 148, 150, 158, 161, 176
  first, 25, 63, 127 (*see also* pregnancy, before first period)
  heavy, 27, 32, 140
  missed, 30–31, 243–45
  painful, 21, 26–30, 34–35, 137, 140, 148, 150
pheromones, 68
Pill, the (*see* contraceptive pill)
pimples (*see* acne)
Planned Parenthood Federation of America, 127, 206, 208, 267
plastic surgery, 37, 46, 48–50, 52, 99
police, 226, 235–38
pornography, 86–87, 96, 102–03, 105, 111, 225, 227, 241
positions, sexual, 217, 252, 253–54, 255
pre-ejaculate, 20, 127 (*see also* ejaculation)
pregnancy, 118, 154, 205, 220, 242–51,
  257, 264–65, 267 (*see also* contraception)
  before first period, 25, 127, 200, 211 (*see also* periods, first)
  prevention of, 58, 120, 125–55, 190, 199, 211, 265
  teenage, 96, 126, 242, 246–49
  tests for, 31, 207, 244
premature ejaculation, 254–55 (*see also* ejaculation)
premenstrual syndrome (PMS), 28–30, 137, 140
prenatal care, 207, 243, 245, 247–48
pressure to have sex, 100, 106, 111, 117–124, 184–85, 187–91, 213, 224, 257 (*see also* peer presure; saying no to sex)
proctitis, 169
progesterone (*see* hormones)
progestin (*see* hormones)
progestin-only pill (*see* contraceptive pill)
prostate gland, 19
prostitution, 103
puberty, 3–20, 21, 23, 44, 188 (*see also* adolescence)
pubic bones, 10
pubic hair, 5, 7–8, 10, 11, 15, 169–71 (*see also* hair)
pubic lice, 157, 169–71

QueerAmerica, 263–64

rape, 224, 230–39, 266
Rape, Abuse & Incest National Network, The, 266
readiness (*see* sexual intercourse, readiness for)
regrets, 96, 104, 106, 115, 116–21, 123–124, 190, 197, 205, 223 (*see also* guilt)
relationships, 36, 67–83, 86, 87, 95, 98, 105, 107–12, 181, 204, 246, 249
  sex and, 96–97, 101, 104, 119–21, 124, 128, 187–210, 214, 219–20, 232–33, 256–57
  successful, 100, 106, 192
religion, 69, 98, 104, 105, 108–09, 118, 121, 126
reproductive organs, 85
  damage to, 159, 176
  female, 3, 5, 12, 21–24, 157
  male, 3, 17–20
respect, 96, 111, 112, 121, 188, 189, 191, 257
Rohypnol, 233 (*see also* drugs, date-rape)
role-playing, 202

SafeTeens.com, 266
safety, 224, 238–41, 265–66
saying no to sex, 118, 202, 204–05, 220–21, 232, 256 (*see also* pressure to have sex; waiting to have sex)
scabies, 157, 171–72
school, 100–101
scrotum, 16, 17
sebum, 8
self-esteem, 36, 41, 53–56, 81, 232 (*see also* body image; confidence)
semen, 14, 17, 19–20, 134, 160, 167, 253
Sex, Etc., 265
sex and the law (*see* laws)
sex appeal (*see* attraction)
sex drive, 91, 99, 182, 183–84, 186
sex education, 100–101
sexual abuse, 93–94, 123, 224, 226–30, 236, 260, 266
sexual assault, 224, 230–38
sexual chemistry (*see* attraction)
sexual contact, 30–31, 84, 103, 129, 157–58, 163, 200 (*see also* touching)
sexual feelings, 4, 5, 84, 89, 92, 101, 118–19, 219–20
sexual harassment, 224, 225–26
sexual health, 31, 115, 135, 156, 157, 193, 206, 208–10, 265, 267
sexual intercourse, 10, 30–31, 35, 84, 87, 105, 162, 214–23, 252, 253, 254–57 (*see also* first-time sex)
    with older men, 229–30
    readiness for, 115–24, 125, 190, 195, 202, 204, 221
    words for, 200
sexuality, 84–94
sexually transmitted diseases (STDs), 58, 118, 154, 205, 206, 207, 216, 235, 256
    protection against, 120, 128, 129, 132, 135–36, 138–39, 141, 143, 145, 146, 148, 149, 150, 190, 199, 200, 205, 212, 253, 254, 267
    symptoms of, 156–79
    testing for, 156–58, 200, 202, 207, 208–10, 214, 253
sexual organs (*see* reproductive organs)
sexual orientation, 92–93 (*see also* homosexuals)
shape (*see* body size and shape)
shaving, 7, 8, 63, 171 (*see also* hair)
side effects, 132, 138, 140, 143, 148, 150, 153
single parents, 96, 246–47, 248
"69," 253–54 (*see also* oral sex)
skank, 186
skin, 8, 15, 149–50, 162, 163, 171,

177, 209, 215 (*see also* acne; foreskin)
    color of, 11, 13–14, 17, 20, 27, 37, 45, 46, 47, 166
slut, 186, 201
smear test (*see* cervical smear)
smells, 9, 16, 33, 34, 57–58, 68, 158, 173, 174, 175, 177
smoking, 138, 140, 142, 174, 247
sperm, 17, 19–20, 24, 30, 127–28, 131, 133, 212, 242, 243
spermicide, 130, 132, 135, 144, 145, 146
stimulation, sexual, 11–14, 85, 90, 91, 121, 221–22, 254 (*see also* foreplay; masturbation)
Stop Bullying Now!, 225, 260
stopping (*see* saying no to sex)
straights (*see* heterosexuals)
stress, 27, 30, 163
sweat, 9, 16, 58, 71, 167
symptoms, 137, 158–59, 165, 209 (*see also* breasts, soreness in; genitals, soreness in; pain)
    bleeding, 158, 161, 175
    diarrhea, 34, 142, 147
    discharge, 25, 47, 58, 158, 160–61, 165, 169, 173, 174, 177, 209
    dizziness, 27, 34, 153
    fever, 34, 162, 168, 175
    itchiness, 57, 58, 157, 162, 170, 171, 173, 177
    nausea/vomiting, 28, 34, 42, 138, 142, 147, 153, 239, 243
    pregnancy, 243–44
    rash, 34, 157, 171, 172
    smells, 57–58, 68, 157, 173, 174, 175
    sores, 157, 162–63, 173, 177
    swelling, 25, 161, 168
syphilis, 157, 158, 172–73, 210

talking about sex, 193–210
    to boyfriends, 77–78, 79–82, 181, 192, 199–205, 219–21, 252
    to doctors and other health professionals, 47, 93, 193, 206–10, 243, 244, 247
    to friends, 55, 87, 98, 193, 197–99, 202, 219, 236–37, 251, 252
    to parents, 96–98, 193–96
tampons, 9, 12, 13, 21, 27, 31, 33–35, 60–61, 116, 148, 178
teasing, 57, 100, 187 (*see also* bullying)
teenage motherhood, 96, 246–49
teenage years (*see* adolescence; puberty)
TeensHealth, 264
Teenwire.com, 267
testicles, 15, 17, 19–20, 161, 164, 166, 188–89 (*see also* blue balls)
testosterone (*see* hormones)

thongs, 32, 33
thoughts, 54–55
    sexual, 17, 84, 85, 86, 87, 110
threesome, 252, 256–57
throbbing, 85
thrombosis, 140
thrush, 157, 177–79
Tolerance.org, 260
touching, 119, 157, 253, 256 (*see also*
    sexual contact)
toxic shock syndrome (TSS), 34–35, 60
trichomonas vaginalis (TV), 157, 158,
    173
trust, 106, 112, 120, 187, 205, 228
two-timing, 82

underage sex, 101–02, 105–06, 108,
    229–30
under-sixteens
    abortion and, 250-51
    contraception for, 116, 207
    pregnancy and, 245
    regrets of, 118, 205
    sex and, 84, 96, 105–06, 108, 110,
        116, 200
    sexual assault of, 229–30
urethra, 10, 11–12, 14, 169, 173, 175
urination, 58, 158, 160–61, 162, 165-66,
    169, 173, 175, 178, 243
U.S. Equal Employment Opportunity
    Commission, 226
uterus (*see* womb)

vagina, 10, 11, 12–13, 21–22, 35, 59,
    60–61, 84, 85, 116, 119, 122, 201,
    212, 214, 221, 222–23, 231, 253, 254
    bleeding from, 137, 140, 141, 148,
        149, 158, 161, 176
    contraception involving, 127, 128,
        130, 131, 134, 144–45, 209,
        212
    discharge from, 23–24, 25, 33, 58,
        158, 160, 165, 167, 169, 173,
        174, 177
    inflammation of, 169, 177
    lubrication of, 12, 217, 218, 253,
        257
values, 69, 95–104, 109, 118, 121
vibrators, 91, 252, 254
virginity, 13, 115, 116–17, 157–58, 209,
    212
    loss of, 35, 100–01, 106, 116–18,
        121, 212, 218
vitamins, 27, 29, 60
voices, changes in, 5, 16–17
vulva, 9–13

waiting to have sex, 115–24, 187–91,
    195, 202, 204–05, 257 (*see also* say-
        ing no to sex)
warts (*see* genital warts)
waxing, 7–8, 63
weight, 6, 15, 36, 38–43, 57, 63–64,
    138, 143, 150 (*see also* body size
    and shape)
wet dreams, 19–20 (*see also* dreams)
whitlows, 161–62
withdrawal method, 127–28, 242
womb, 12, 21–24, 26–27, 157, 242–43,
    249, 253 (*see also* cancer, uterine;
    cervix)
    contraception effects on, 136, 139,
        141, 144–49, 151–52, 155
yeast infections, 58, 157, 177–79

Tina Radziszewicz has worked as a freelance writer and editor for more than twenty national women's, teenage, film, and television magazines since 1988, and she has been an advice columnist for the past twelve years. Her commitment to helping people fulfill their potential led her to train as a psychotherapist, and she has been running a private practice since 2000.

Tina lives in South London with her husband, Mark, her son, Alex, a pair of unusually wise cats, and a ghost in her attic (whom the cats refuse to take on). This is her first book.